STRONGER TH[illegible]ER MENOPAUSE BOOK FOR WOMEN ATHLETE

A Woman's Guide to Wisdom within, Proper Diet and Healthier version of yourself in Menopause to Rule Your Life Again

Dr. Eulalia Lark

1

Introduction

Thank you for visiting "Stronger Than Ever Menopause Book For Women Athlete." This book is your travel companion as you begin on a life-changing trip that brings together menopause and physical activity. You've already shown resiliency, dedication and a desire for pushing your limits as a female athlete. This manual will equip you with the expertise you need to confidently navigate the current phase of life while maximizing both your athletic performance and psychological health as you now approach the distinct opportunities and challenges that menopause goodies.

This book's each chapter are carefully written to discuss a different aspect of menopause and how this impacts female athletes. We'll cover everything, from figuring out how your body is affected by hormone changes to maximizing you're eating and exercise plans.

You've been training, battling it out, and achieving amazing achievements for years. Your body has been an effective weapon for success, empowering you to succeed in the sport of your choice. Your body is now going under a new stage of evolution as you enter the menopause. It's time to make adjustments to the changes put on by menopause, just as you have done in the past when modifying your workout plans and techniques.

Menopause is a remarkable stage of life to treasure, not a challenge to get over. This book provides your road map, guiding you through the rough patches with insight, self-compassion, and a dedication to maintaining your athletic identity. You'll discover beneficial advice in these pages to help you succeed whether you're a professional athlete, weekend warrior, or someone who just enjoys the thrill of movement.

So, let's continue this trip together. By the moment that you finish this book, you'll not only have useful tips but also an updated feeling of empowerment as you continue to update what it means to be a tough and stubborn female athlete.

Menopause is a natural and inevitable phase in a woman's life, marking the end of her reproductive years. Typically occurring in the late 40s to early 50s, menopause is a significant biological event that signifies the cessation of menstrual cycles. This transition is a normal part of the aging process and is influenced by various hormonal changes within the female body.

One of the primary hallmarks of menopause is the decline in the production of key reproductive hormones, such as estrogen and progesterone. These hormonal fluctuations play a crucial role in the regulation of the menstrual cycle and impact various physiological processes throughout a woman's reproductive years. As menopause approaches, the ovaries gradually reduce their hormone production, leading to the cessation of ovulation and menstruation.

The symptoms of menopause can vary widely among women, both in terms of intensity and duration. While some women may experience minimal discomfort, others may undergo more pronounced physical and emotional changes. Common symptoms include hot flashes, night sweats, mood swings, and changes in sleep patterns. These symptoms can have a significant impact on a woman's overall well-being and may require personalized approaches for effective management.

Beyond the physical manifestations, menopause also represents a psychological and emotional adjustment for many women. The end of fertility can evoke a range of feelings, including a sense of loss or liberation. Additionally, the hormonal fluctuations associated with menopause can influence mood and cognitive function, contributing to challenges such as memory lapses and difficulty concentrating.

It is essential to recognize menopause as a natural and transformative phase, acknowledging the diversity of experiences among women. While the biological aspects are paramount, the emotional and psychological dimensions of this life stage are equally significant. As women navigate through this transitional period, they may seek support from healthcare professionals, friends, and family to manage the changes and embrace the next chapter of their lives. Understanding and addressing the multifaceted aspects of menopause can contribute to a more positive and empowered experience for women entering this phase of their journey.

PERIMENOPAUSE

Perimenopause is a transitional phase that occurs in a woman's life leading up to menopause. Menopause is defined as the point when a woman has not had a menstrual period for 12 consecutive months. Perimenopause typically starts several years before menopause and is marked by hormonal fluctuations and changes in the reproductive system.

During perimenopause, the ovaries gradually produce less estrogen, the primary female sex hormone. Estrogen plays a crucial role in regulating the menstrual cycle and maintaining various aspects of reproductive health. As estrogen levels fluctuate, women may experience a range of physical and emotional symptoms.

One of the first signs of perimenopause is often changes in the menstrual cycle. Periods may become irregular, with variations in the length of the cycle and the amount of flow.

MENOPAUSE

Menopause marks a specific moment in a woman's life the day she realizes, usually after a year without menstruation if she has been keeping tabs on it. While the average age for menopause is around 51 or 52, certain factors such as premature ovarian failure can bring about menopause as early as 40. On the other hand, some women experience late-onset menopause, entering this phase between the ages of 55 and 60.

For individuals uncertain about their menopausal status, the picoAMH Elisa diagnostic test can provide clarity and either confirm or dispel any uncertainties. Once menopause is verified, the subsequent stage is referred to as postmenopause, denoting the hormonal state that will persist for the rest of a woman's life.

POSTMENOPAUSE

Postmenopause is a stage in a woman's life that follows the cessation of menstrual periods, marking the end of the reproductive phase. It typically begins around the age of 50, although the timing can vary among individuals. Unlike menopause, which is the immediate period when a woman stops menstruating, postmenopause encompasses the years that follow, extending throughout the rest of a woman's life.

At the core of postmenopause are profound hormonal shifts that significantly impact a woman's body and overall well-being. The primary hormones involved are estrogen and progesterone, which played crucial roles in the reproductive processes during the fertile years. These hormones, produced by the ovaries, not only regulated the menstrual cycle but also influenced various physiological functions, including bone health, cardiovascular health, and the maintenance of reproductive tissues.

As a woman enters postmenopause, the ovaries gradually reduce their production of estrogen and progesterone. This decline is a natural and expected part of the aging process, leading to a new hormonal landscape that requires adaptation. The hormonal fluctuations experienced during postmenopause can have far-reaching effects on different systems within the body, influencing physical, emotional, and cognitive aspects of a woman's life.

Understanding the intricate interplay between hormonal changes and their impacts during postmenopause is essential for both women and healthcare professionals. It allows for a more comprehensive approach to managing the challenges associated with this life stage, promoting overall health and well-being. Exploring the nuanced effects of these hormonal shifts without delving into specific symptoms provides a foundation for further discussion on the various dimensions of postmenopausal health and the potential strategies for managing this transformative phase of a woman's life.

SYMTOMPS OF MENOPAUSE

Menopause is a natural biological process that marks the end of a woman's reproductive years. It typically occurs in the late 40s or early 50s, but the age at which menopause occurs can vary. The transition leading up to menopause is called perimenopause, and it can last for several years. During this time, women may experience a variety of symptoms as their bodies adjust to the hormonal changes. Here are some common symptoms of menopause:

Irregular Menstrual Cycles: One of the earliest signs of perimenopause is changes in the menstrual cycle. Periods may become irregular, with variations in the length of the cycle and the flow.

Hot Flashes and Night Sweats: Sudden feelings of intense heat, usually concentrated around the face and upper body, are known as hot flashes. Night sweats are episodes of sweating during sleep that can disrupt sleep patterns.

Vaginal Changes: The decrease in estrogen levels can lead to changes in the vaginal tissues, resulting in dryness, itching, and discomfort during sexual intercourse. This condition is known as vaginal atrophy.

Sleep Disturbances: Many women experience difficulties with sleep during menopause. This can include insomnia, difficulty falling asleep, or waking up frequently during the night.

Mood Swings: Hormonal fluctuations can contribute to mood swings, irritability, and increased susceptibility to stress. Some women may also experience symptoms of anxiety or depression.

Weight Gain: Changes in hormonal balance can contribute to changes in body composition, with some women noticing an increase in abdominal fat.

Joint and Muscle Pain: Menopause can be associated with joint and muscle pain, often due to a decrease in estrogen levels.

Memory and Concentration Issues: Some women report difficulties with memory and concentration during menopause, often referred to as "menopausal fog" or "brain fog."

Changes in Libido: Fluctuating hormone levels can affect sexual desire. Some women may experience a decrease in libido, while others may find an increase.

Urinary Changes: The decline in estrogen levels can lead to changes in the urinary tract, resulting in increased frequency of urination and an increased risk of urinary tract infections.

2

Impact of Hormonal Changes

The field of hormone therapy has continuously evolved since the introduction of estrogen therapy in 1949 and the advent of birth control pills in the 1960s. These pills provided women with a convenient solution to navigate daily life without being mindful of natural hormonal and fertility patterns. Unfortunately, this led to the pathologizing of these natural rhythms, fostering the belief that synthetic hormones are superior to the "unpredictable" ones produced naturally in our bodies. This mindset extended to hormone replacement therapy (HRT), viewing the female body as deficient and in need of correction.

Today, there are more respectful options that align with the body's wisdom. A shift in thinking emphasizes personalized hormone levels instead of a one-size-fits-all approach. Hormone therapy (HT) is now the preferred term over HRT. Understanding the evolution of views on hormones and therapy requires a brief historical perspective.

Advocating estrogen pills to counteract the perceived decline in a woman's body at menopause. This reflected a cultural devaluation of female bodies ingrained in medical practice. The subsequent 1970s studies revealing the increased risk of uterine cancer with estrogen use and adverse effects of birth control pills caused a decline in Premarin sales.

Despite this, studies in the 1980s and '90s suggested cardiovascular benefits of estrogen, reviving Premarin's popularity. However, a link between estrogen supplementation and breast cancer emerged, challenging the prevailing belief in the cardiovascular benefits. The Women's Health Initiative studies in 2002 dealt a significant blow to the perceived benefits of long-term Prempro use, revealing increased risks of breast cancer, heart attacks, strokes, and blood clots.

This revelation prompted a paradigm shift in the cultural perception of hormone therapy, with women discontinuing its use. Subsequent studies in the mid-2000s highlighted nuanced findings, showing reduced heart attack risk in younger HT users but increased risks for older women, especially after ten years post-menopause.

In conclusion, the journey of understanding menopause and hormone therapy dispels the notion of a universal, indefinite solution. The evolving science of hormone therapy, acknowledged by the North American Menopause Society, emphasizes benefits close to menopause, acknowledging diminishing benefits in older women and over time since menopause. While hormone therapy presents tangible benefits, there is a need to balance them with potential risks and side effects, fostering an individualized approach to women's health.

NATURE'S OPTIMAL DESIGN: BIOIDENTICAL HORMONES

Bioidentical hormones, unlike Premarin, Provera, and Prempro, closely mirror the hormones naturally found in the female body. Although synthesized from soybeans or yams in the lab, they precisely replicate human hormones, making them bioidentical. This term is more accurate than "natural," which can be ambiguous.

Bioidentical hormones offer more physiologic effects consistent with normal biochemistry, minimizing unpredictable side effects at low replacement doses compared to synthetic non-bioidentical hormones. Ongoing large-scale clinical trials, such as ELITE and KEEPS, are exploring the benefits of bioidentical hormones in reducing atherosclerosis and heart disease risk in menopausal women.

To reap the benefits of bioidentical hormone therapy, one must abandon the notion of a universal solution. The decision to use hormone therapy varies among women, with some needing it for a short duration and others opting for a longer term.

The inconsistency and market influence in hormone therapy science prompt a reliance on inner wisdom and intuition in decision-making—an embodiment of feminine wisdom. Moving beyond Premarin, equine estrogens with potential side effects, bioidentical estrogens at individualized low doses may offer relief without the same carcinogenic impact on breast tissue, though long-term studies are lacking.

While long-term studies are costly, prescribing bioidentical hormone therapy for short-term symptom relief is favored by many clinicians, especially as awareness of physiologic alternatives grows amid shifting views on Premarin and Prempro. The evolving nature of this process underscores the importance of making hormone choices in alignment with personal guidance.

Research Summary of Hormone Therapy

Estrogen offers various benefits during menopause

Hot Flashes Relief: Estrogen is highly effective in alleviating hot flashes, with noticeable results in up to four weeks.

Urinary Tract Health: Local application of estrogen may decrease the risk of urinary tract infection. However, systemic estrogen increases the likelihood of stress urinary incontinence.

Skin Improvement: Whether administered systemically or topically, estrogen enhances skin thickness, boosts the collagen layer, and reduces wrinkles in women with low estrogen levels.

Depression: Estrogen may have an antidepressive effect in some women, but it shouldn't be the primary treatment. Synthetic progestins may induce depression in certain cases, and menopause itself isn't linked to increased depression.

Sexual Function: Estrogen, applied either systemically or topically, eliminates vaginal dryness and thinning, enhancing sexual function. Some studies suggest it may also increase sexual desire.

Cognition Support: While estrogen doesn't improve established dementia, research indicates that starting hormone therapy, especially with the estradiol patch, soon after menopause may moderately protect against cognitive decline.

Osteoporosis Prevention: Estrogen has a well-documented positive impact on bone density, comparable to bisphosphonates like Fosamax. It reduces fracture risk, likely through a different mechanism than SERMs or bisphosphonates.

Heart and Blood Vessels: Controversial findings exist regarding estrogen's cardiovascular effects. While past studies showed conflicting data, current research, including the ELITE and KEEPS studies, aims to provide clearer insights. As of now, authorities don't recommend estrogen for preventing chronic diseases based on the latest evidence from the North American Menopause Society.

Neutral Effects of Estrogen

Weight Changes and Insulin Resistance: Estrogen doesn't cause weight gain or affect blood sugar in individuals with diabetes.

Ovarian, Endometrial, and Bowel Cancer: Prolonged estrogen use may increase ovarian cancer risk. Estrogen therapy without progesterone raises endometrial cancer risk, but this risk is eliminated with progesterone. While estrogen decreases colorectal cancer risk, it shouldn't be prescribed solely for this purpose, according to the American College of Obstetrics and Gynecology Hormone Therapy Task Force.

Osteoarthritis: Estrogen has no significant impact, positive or negative, on individuals with osteoarthritis.

Estrogen Risks

Breast Cancer: Multiple studies indicate that estrogen raises breast cancer risk, though the absolute risk with conventional hormone therapy (estrogen plus synthetic progesterone) is low (twenty additional cases per 10,000 women over five years). Notably, well-designed studies, including a large-scale one comparing bioidentical and synthetic hormones, show significantly lower breast cancer risk with natural hormones.

Ovarian Cancer: Estrogen-only hormone therapy increases ovarian cancer risk by 63%, while any hormone therapy raises the risk by 29%, as per the European Prospective Investigation into Cancer and Nutrition.

Pancreatitis and Gallstones: High triglyceride levels elevate the risk of pancreatitis with oral estrogen use. All women face an increased risk of gallstones and biliary tract issues with estrogen use.

Blood Clots and Stroke: Estrogen doubles the risk of blood clots and pulmonary embolism, especially in the first year of therapy and notably in smokers and older women. Unopposed estrogen also increases stroke risk, according to randomized trials.

Stable Approach of Personalized Bioidentical Hormone

A variety of bioidentical hormones, available by prescription from formulary pharmacies, can be tailored to an individual's needs. Dosages are adjustable based on test results and symptoms, ensuring optimal hormone levels. This approach, standard for thyroid hormone, has recently been extended to sex hormones. Creating a bioidentical hormone regimen is possible using preparations from conventional pharmacies; awareness of bioidentical brands is crucial.

These personalized hormones can be taken orally, transdermally, or vaginally, with the transdermal route being physiologically superior due to direct bloodstream entry, enabling lower doses. Oral preparations necessitate absorption from the gut and liver processing, associated with increased clotting factors and heightened risks.

Popularly, a prescription can combine bioidentical estrogens (estradiol, estrone, estriol), progesterone, and an androgen (DHEA or testosterone), forming a lotion or cream applied to the skin. Research affirms that transdermal regimens effectively provide hormone levels, protect the uterine lining, and offer relief for perimenopausal symptoms.

Why Synthetic Hormones Proliferate

Economic incentives drive the prevalence of synthetic hormones. Bioidentical hormones lack patentability, dissuading pharmaceutical investment in research and development. Synthetic hormones, patentable due to molecular alterations, may retain some natural hormone activity but pose unknown risks. Trusting nature's wisdom is contrasted with synthetic experimentation spanning only fifty years.

Considerations on Birth Control Pills

While birth control pills are convenient for managing perimenopausal symptoms, their synthetic composition masks natural hormonal rhythms. Advocating early and prolonged pill use for perceived health benefits contradicts the potential side effects and disconnect from natural cycles. Awareness of available alternatives is crucial, allowing women to make choices aligning with their well-being.

HORMONE BASICS: CRUCIAL KNOWLEDGE FOR WOMEN

Understanding hormone therapy extends beyond estrogen; it encompasses other ovarian hormones like progesterone and androgens such as testosterone. Women's needs vary; some may be comfortable without supplemental hormones, while others may require progesterone or a combination of all three. Familiarity with their original roles in the body and responses to dropping levels aids in making informed hormone therapy decisions.

Estrogen Insights

Estrogen, traditionally the primary prescription for menopausal symptoms, includes three natural compounds: estradiol, estrone, and estriol. Estriol, highest during pregnancy, exhibits milder effects on breast and uterine tissue. Locally applied estriol effectively addresses urogenital symptoms. Perimenopausal symptoms often link more to progesterone deficiency than estrogen. Estrogen's role changes after menopause, with estrone becoming predominant, likely contributing to heart, brain, and bone health.

Symptoms due to Deficiency of Estrogen

- Hot flashes
- Mood swings
- Headaches, migraines
- Night sweats
- Mental fuzziness
- Vaginal dryness
- Vaginal/bladder infections
- Thinning of vaginal walls
- Incontinence; recurrent urinary tract infections

Symptoms Due to Excess of Estrogen

- Depression
- Bilateral, pounding headache
- Nausea, vomiting
- Recurrent vaginal yeast infections

- Yellow-tinged skin
- Breast swelling/tenderness
- Excessive vaginal bleeding
- Bloating
- Leg cramps

Designer Estrogens: SERMs Unveiled

Selective estrogen receptor modulators (SERMs), synthetic drugs like tamoxifen and raloxifene, selectively modulate estrogen effects in different tissues. Tamoxifen blocks breast cell estrogen receptors, maintaining positive effects on bone, uterine tissue, and the cardiovascular system. Raloxifene, prescribed for osteoporosis, offers less bone protection than estrogen. Concerns surround SERMs' unnatural origin and potential long-term risks, including Alzheimer's disease. Documented side effects and incomplete knowledge caution against prolonged SERM use. Bioidentical hormones or alternative options are preferable unless no other choice exists.

Understanding Progesterone Changes

The initial hormonal shift signaling menopause often begins with a decline in progesterone levels, manifesting symptoms years before menopause is suspected. The intricate balance between progesterone and estrogen falters, resulting in estrogen dominance, displaying symptoms of both progesterone deficiency and relative estrogen excess.

Progesterone Functions and Sources

Progesterone, primarily originating from the ovaries throughout a woman's life, serves a crucial role in preparing and maintaining the uterus for pregnancy. It also acts as a uterine muscle relaxant, preventing premature contractions. Beyond reproduction, progesterone influences brain function, inducing calmness and promoting restful sleep. As women age, the likelihood of follicles failing to ovulate increases, leading to a gradual progesterone deficiency.

Symptoms of Progesterone Deficiency

- Premenstrual migraine
- Irregular or excessively heavy periods
- PMS-like symptoms

Symptoms of Excess Progesterone

- Depression
- Sleepiness
- Drowsiness

Bioidentical Progesterone: Alleviating Symptoms

Bioidentical progesterone supplementation addresses both progesterone deficiency and estrogen excess symptoms, restoring the body's equilibrium. Evidence suggests that combining estrogen therapy with an appropriate dose of progesterone mitigates the risk of uterine cancer. Studies comparing bioidentical and synthetic hormones reveal lower associated breast cancer risks with bioidentical hormones. Additionally, natural progesterone exhibits promise in relieving midlife chest pain, and ongoing research explores its potential in heart drugs for women.

Advantages of Progesterone Supplementation

Supplemental progesterone offers unique advantages, such as conversion into other hormones as needed. It can transform into testosterone, increase DHEA levels, and under specific circumstances, metabolize into estrogen. Progesterone cream, available over the counter, is a popular choice, offering flexibility in application. Prescription options include gel or oral micronized forms. Research indicates that even small amounts of topical progesterone are absorbed by the body, emphasizing its efficacy.

Note: Progesterone supplementation should be considered cautiously, especially in cases of depression triggered by synthetic progestins. Chasteberry (Vitex agnus-castus) may be explored for natural progesterone increase in sensitive individuals.

Challenges with Synthetic Hormones

The use of synthetic progestin presents a distinct set of issues. A widely prescribed progestin, medroxyprogesterone acetate (MPA), along with others like norethindrone, norgestrel, and norgestimate, tends to induce or exacerbate various symptoms (refer to the list on page 174). This reinforces my caution against hormone therapy programs incorporating synthetic progestins. The 2002 Women's Health Initiative

(WHI) findings link synthetic progestins to increased risks of strokes, heart disease, and breast cancer.

MPA, specifically, has been found to diminish estrogen's positive effects on blood vessels, causing increased vascular resistance, inhibited blood flow, and heightened cerebral artery resistance. A substantial study involving continuous therapy of estrogen plus MPA resulted in a significant rise in myocardial infarction, death from coronary artery disease, and venous thrombosis during the initial two years of treatment.

Recent analysis of WHI data reconfirmed the persistent risk of synthetic hormone therapy, even for women initiating it within ten years of menopause. Although the risk diminishes after six years of use, this duration exceeds the typical period women pursue hormone therapy. Earlier reanalysis from 2006 also suggested adverse effects from synthetic progestin, notably in heart disease risk for women on Prempro. Natural bioidentical progesterone, in contrast, carries no such risks and offers multiple benefits. In the PEPI trial, oral natural progesterone prevented adverse cholesterol effects observed in women on Provera.

Symptoms Induced by Synthetic Progestin:

- Weight gain and bloating
- Moodiness
- Headache
- Depression
- Lack of sexual desire

- Potential narrowing of blood vessels, causing chest pain and reduced heart oxygenation

Case Study: Eve's Experience

Eve, a potter and yoga instructor, faced symptoms like mental fuzziness, dizziness, and headaches during her early forties. Her doctor, based on high FSH levels, diagnosed menopause and prescribed daily Premarin with Provera for the last twelve days of each month. However, Eve's condition worsened, revealing symptoms consistent with estrogen overdose. Intuitively, she ceased estrogen intake and felt relief within twenty-four hours. Subsequent hormone tests identified low progesterone in the early stages of perimenopause. Now using natural progesterone cream, Eve has significantly improved, emphasizing the importance of understanding individual hormonal needs.

Testosterone Dynamics

Testosterone, a hormone produced in the ovaries and adrenal glands, plays a pivotal role in providing assertive energy and fostering sexual drive. It contributes to heightened sexual arousal, increased initiation of sexual activity, enhanced erogenous zone sensitivity, more frequent orgasms, intensified sexual fantasies, and a rise in orgasmic dreams.

While not all women experience a decline in testosterone levels during perimenopause in fact, some may witness an increase certain factor, such as adrenal depletion due to chronic stress or medical interventions like surgical procedures, chemotherapy, radiation, or autoimmune diseases, can lead to a significant drop in testosterone, resulting in symptoms like diminishing libido and overall energy depletion.

Understanding the necessity of confirming testosterone deficiency through saliva or blood testing before considering supplementation is crucial. Some women might encounter a decline in libido due to estrogen deficiency, despite having normal testosterone levels. Hence, testosterone supplementation should only be pursued if a deficiency is confirmed. Many women mistakenly seek testosterone supplementation to rejuvenate their sex lives, emphasizing the importance of accurate testing.

If a deficiency exists, supplementing with bioidentical testosterone or DHEA (dehydroepiandrosterone), an adrenal precursor for testosterone, can offer benefits like heightened sex drive, improved sexual function, increased overall energy, better muscle tone, enhanced mood, and potentially improved bone mineral density. Incorporating testosterone into a vaginal cream can aid in restoring normal vaginal wall thickness and lubrication. However, unnecessary supplementation can lead to overdose, resulting in objectionable symptoms.

Bioidentical testosterone and DHEA are available from formulary pharmacies, ensuring quality and effectiveness. Pharmaceutical-grade DHEA is recommended, and its sublingual form can be taken daily. Testosterone is also available in patch form.

Symptoms of Testosterone Deficiency

- Decreased sense of well-being
- Thinning pubic hair
- Decreased libido
- Impaired sexual function
- Decreased energy overall

Symptoms of Testosterone Overdose

- Increased facial hair growth
- Deepened voice
- Mood disturbances
- Acne, particularly on the face and scalp

NAVIGATING HORMONE THERAPY CHOICES

Deciding whether to embark on hormone therapy (HT) during menopause involves considering various factors such as overall physical health, emotional well-being, spiritual aspects, nutritional status, and lifestyle. These elements influence how secondary hormone production sites cope with the body's changing needs. Some women find reassurance in knowing that perimenopausal symptoms are temporary, opting to experience them without medication. Relaxing and letting go of fears and resistance may also contribute to symptom reduction through the placebo effect, influencing menopausal treatments.

Evaluating Before Committing

Before choosing hormone therapy, conduct an honest self-assessment, considering personal and family medical history. While some women naturally produce sufficient hormones to navigate menopause, others may struggle with biological conversions necessary for hormonal balance. Factors like ovarian removal or chronic stress-induced adrenal depletion can affect hormone levels. Despite recent findings on HT and heart disease, I emphasize progesterone's potential in preventing heart disease. Individual experiences vary, and the decision to use hormone therapy should align with personal goals and preferences.

Given the evolving nature of scientific understanding and medical practices, the wisdom surrounding HT is subject to change. Acknowledging the potential benefits and risks, women experiencing bothersome perimenopausal symptoms may consider trying hormone therapy, monitoring its effects for about a year, and adjusting the dosage accordingly. The decision-making process involves identifying risk factors, understanding cultural influences, and recognizing individual responses to expectations.

Personalizing the Decision-Making Process

I encourage viewing the HT decision as a process rather than a binary choice. Defining goals for hormone therapy is crucial, recognizing that it won't reverse aging but can alleviate physical symptoms and health concerns. A tailored program, with or without hormones, can help manage symptoms, but it won't address underlying relationship issues or stress. Various studies highlight the effectiveness of alternatives like dietary changes, supplements, exercise, and herbs, offering choices beyond hormone therapy. Becoming an active participant in the decision-making process, armed with information and options, allows women to create individualized treatment plans supportive of their unique menopausal journey.

Initiating HT Timing

Dispelling the notion of delaying HT until menopause, the author emphasizes the freedom to start interventions be it hormones, herbs, or lifestyle changes based on individual needs. Perimenopause, marked by heightened symptoms, is a valid period for intervention. For those wary of hormonal risks, especially related to cancer, the author suggests considering bioidentical estrogen at low doses for symptomatic relief during the intrusive phase.

Principles of HT: A Guiding Framework

I have introduced key principles for Hormone Therapy (HT), emphasizing personalized, informed decisions. These principles include establishing natural hormonal levels, replacing only necessary hormones, using minimal effective doses, opting for bioidentical hormones, and supporting HT with a holistic approach, encompassing diet, supplements, and exercise. The overarching goal is not reversal but optimization of comfort and overall health.

The Timing Hypothesis: Unravelling Hormone Therapy Mysteries

Scientists explore the "timing hypothesis," investigating why HT's effects vary based on initiation age. The hypothesis extends to heart health, brain health, cancer risks, osteoporosis, and mood disorders. A January 2010 symposium highlighted this concept, focusing on the "Window of Opportunity of Estrogen Therapy for Neuroprotection." The age-related impact lies in estrogen's ability to unlock positive effects in a healthy brain, contrasting with potential harm in aging or Alzheimer's-afflicted brains. The complexity of determining brain health at HT initiation underscores the ongoing research in this groundbreaking area.

A HINT OF HORMONAL BALANCE

Suppose you're contemplating hormone therapy, experiencing hot flashes before periods, and occasional night sweats. Testing your hormone levels approximately a week before your period offers insights into peak progesterone, estrogen, and testosterone levels. These measurements establish a baseline for future hormone therapy.

Depending on your levels, begin supplementing the lowest hormone, often progesterone, potentially accompanied by estrogen. A 2 percent natural progesterone skin cream, available over the counter, could suffice. Administer it for two weeks before your period, then take a break. Adjust the duration based on symptom relief.

For low estrogen or intense hot flashes, start with the lowest available estrogen level. Prescription-only estrogen, whether in patches or pills, requires professional guidance. Divigel, a natural estrogen gel, offers a convenient alternative, with varying strengths. Studies indicate significant symptom reduction with the lowest dose after five weeks.

If using estrogen, ensure sufficient progesterone to prevent uterine lining buildup. A 2 percent progesterone skin cream might suffice, or prescription options like Crinone vaginal gel or Prometrium capsules could be necessary. Many healthcare providers embrace bioidentical natural hormones, working with compounding pharmacies for personalized prescriptions.

Choose accredited formulary pharmacies for quality assurance. Some health plans cover these prescriptions, so advocate for coverage. Confirm your doctor's openness to individualized natural hormone approaches before appointments. If not, educate them or seek practitioners familiar with this approach, often found among nurse practitioners.

HORMONE DURATION DILEMMA

Deciding how long to continue hormone therapy hinges on its purpose and concurrent health strategies. If estrogen was initially adopted for bone health, incorporating regular weight training might allow tapering off while maintaining bone density. Conversely, individuals at osteoporosis risk due to a sedentary lifestyle, steroid use, or smoking should prioritize bone health with measures like a low-acid diet and optimizing vitamin D levels.

For short-term relief of menopausal symptoms like hot flashes, most women turn to hormones, herbs, or a combination. This contrasts with those focused on preventing long-term issues such as osteoporosis or preserving sexual function. Menopausal symptoms typically peak over five to ten years, subsiding naturally thereafter.

Despite concerns, some women, like a sixty-two-year-old who consulted for advice, have taken bioidentical hormones for well over a decade. Feeling revitalized on a daily dose of oral estrogen and 100 mg progesterone, she's hesitant to discontinue due to potential spaciness and urinary incontinence without them. While acknowledging the potential risk, the recommendation is to continue based on enhanced quality of life. Decisions around hormone therapy's duration must be tailored to individual circumstances, weighing present well-being against remote possibilities.

Transitioning from Hormone Therapy

If you're considering discontinuing Hormone Therapy (HT), avoid abrupt cessation. Opt for a gradual and slow weaning process, allowing your body sufficient time to adapt. Consider the following sample weaning schedule:

- Week one: Omit Sunday's pill
- Week two: Omit Sunday and Tuesday
- Week three: Omit Sunday, Tuesday, and Thursday
- Week four: Omit Sunday, Tuesday, Thursday, and Saturday
- Week five: Omit Sunday, Tuesday, Thursday, Friday, and Saturday
- Week six: Complete cessation of hormones

3

The Menopausal Fitness Equation – To Exercise or Not?

Menopause is commonly associated with a range of health complaints, including hot flashes, urinary disorders, joint pain and psychological distress. Women reporting menopausal symptoms are generally of overall poorer health. Serious chronic conditions such as osteoporosis and cardiovascular diseases are more likely to occur after menopause than before. In this respect physical activity has a positive impact on bone density in menopausal women. For example, greater physical activity within 4 life domains, of, sport, active living, home, and work was associated with higher peak femoral neck strength relative to load in 1919 menopausal women. Moreover, physical activity has a positive effect in the tibial cartilage of the knee during menopause.

It is clear that there are many benefits of exercise on bone, cardiovascular, metabolic, diabetes, cancer, longevity, psychological wellbeing and overall quality of life. Hence, it is appropriate for women to be physically active throughout the menopausal transition and afterwards.

TO EXERCISE

It is believed that loss of estrogen levels in women to be the main cause of the symptoms associated with menopause. According to the Centre for Disease Control and Prevention, regular exercise helps relieve stress, enhances overall quality of life, and reduces weight gain and muscle loss, the most frequent side effects of menopause. It is recommended that at least 150 minutes of aerobic activity and 75 minutes of vigorous activity to be undertaken per week for cardiovascular health. In addition, strength training should be included in order to build bone and muscle strength, aid in body fat burn and increase in metabolism, also important factors during menopause.

For example, in a group of menopausal women aged 55-72 who were involved in an exercise program, of 3 hours per week for 12 months, experienced significantly improved physical and mental health and overall quality of life compared to those who were sedentary. More importantly a higher proportion of those who did not participate in the exercise regime reported menopause symptoms (58% reporting symptoms at the beginning of the study compared to 68% at the end of the study), compared to a significant lower reporting in those participating in the exercise study (50% reporting prior to the study compared to 37% at the end of the study). Exercise is therefore considered an important factor to alleviate menopause symptoms. The woman's ability to choose their preferred physical activity increases the likelihood that they will adhere to exercise as a treatment method.

Exercise appears to be a cost-effective alternative with few known side effects. Most importantly, women with greater levels of physical activity report improvements in mental and physical aspects of quality of life. Such improvements can even be achieved with low intensity aerobic activity, such as walking and dancing.

Benefits to vasomotor symptoms

The years leading up to menopause, during menopause and early postmenopause, women experience vasomotor related symptoms such as, hot flashes, night sweats and sleep disturbances. Symptoms could be so severe that the overall quality of life of a woman is severely affected. HRT has been shown to alleviate such symptoms but as indicated can have serious side effects. Lifestyle modification interventions, including structured exercise and physical activity, have the potential to reduce vasomotor menopausal symptoms. In fact, in the longitudinal Melbourne Women's Midlife Health Project, in which 438 women were followed over 8 years, those who exercised every day at baseline were 49% less likely to report hot flashes, and those whose exercise levels decreased were more likely to report hot flashes. Moderate physical activity was associated with decreased objective and subjective hot flashes 24 hours post exercise, although worse reported symptoms were reported in women with lower fitness levels. In a randomised controlled trial, 176 symptomatic sedentary women who were given an aerobic exercise regime 50 minutes 4x per week over 6 months, reported a decrease in the frequency of hot flashes. In 3201 women aged 42-52 years old, monitored yearly for 8 years, hot flashes were associated with higher cholesterol, triglyceride and apolipoprotein levels, and in 3075 women, there was a strong correlation between hot flashes and insulin resistance. Physical activity has positive associations in reducing cholesterol, triglycerides, apolipoprotein and glucose levels, and, is associated with reducing hot flash symptoms.

Finally, sleep quality has also been found to be better in menopausal women who are physically active. For example, physically active women have favourable sleep characteristics with fewer awakenings during the night and improved quality of sleep.

Benefits to psychological symptoms

In the years leading up to, and during menopause, many women report symptoms of, depression (unhappiness, irritability, tearfulness, lack of energy) or anxiety (mood swings, insomnia, heart palpitations, panic attacks, forgetfulness or problems with focus and concentration). Studies have found that exercise participation results in lower perception of symptom severity. These findings add to the evidence suggesting that exercise moderates the psychological symptoms associated with menopause. The effects of exercise in reducing psychological symptoms have been widely reported. A study including Australian midlife women, noted, that exercise was beneficial for somatic and psychological symptoms including depression and anxiety, but not for vasomotor symptoms or sexual function. Likewise, in a group of Korean women, those who were depressed experienced more menopausal symptoms than women who were not depressed, and those who exercised on a regular basis, were less depressed and less symptomatic than those who were not physically active.

Exercise as an intervention has also been shown to have a positive impact on menopausal symptoms, depression and quality of life. Providing mental distraction and social interaction are some of the explanations provided for the psychological benefits associated with exercise participation.

Habitual physical activities, those that are part of the participant's lifestyle, such as, walking, cycling, gardening and work-related physical activities of no more than 60 minutes per day, have also been found to have a favourable effect on menopause symptoms and quality of life. They improve mood and enhance psychological functioning. In a cross-sectional study of 151 regular physically activity women the total Greene score and psychological sub-score were found to be improved. Similarly, in 60 postmenopausal women, those in the exercise group reported improvements in depression and anxiety compared to a control group. Overall, an immediate bout of exercise and regular participation is associated with improved psychological functioning in menopausal women.

Benefits to somatic symptoms

Somatic symptoms are those related to the body, which includes muscle and joint pains, numbness or tingling in the extremities or elsewhere, dizziness, headaches and shortness of breath. The health 2000 study in Finnish women reported that physically active women reported significantly fewer somatic symptoms and pain compared to women that were not physically active. Eight years later those that remained physically active exhibited improved quality of life compared to those who were not physically active. Physical activity was also found to improve somatic symptoms in a study of 370 Brazilian women. In addition, in a large cross-sectional study in British women, somatic symptoms were 28% lower among active women. Similarly, in a longitudinal study of 3,300 Australian women, increase in physical activity was associated with fewer somatic symptoms. In the Women's Health Across the Nation (SWAN) study, in over 7 years follow-up, it was noted that physically active women experienced less bodily pain over time during the menopause transition. Likewise, in a 3-year longitudinal study of over 2,400 women from SWAN demonstrated that women who were more physically active at midlife experience less bodily pain over time. This suggests that physical activity positively influences the somatic symptoms in menopausal women and increases overall quality of life.

Benefits to sexual symptoms

As a result of estrogen deprivation during the menopause transition the woman's sexual drive and functioning decreases. Symptoms of vaginal dryness or thinning of the wall, sexual dysfunction or discomfort are common. In a study of 42 postmenopausal women, divided into 2 groups of aerobic or resistance exercise programs of 3 days per week for 8 weeks, no effects were noted for urogenital complaints and sexual symptoms. However, in a cross-sectional study of 151 women who were physical activity, reported improved sexual symptoms. Recently, in 273 Iranian women, a negative significant relation was observed between sexual problems and vaginal dryness and the level of physical activity. The findings with regard to exercise and sexual functioning are equivocal. In addition, this is an area which requires further examination.

OR, NOT TO EXERCISE

Not all studies have provided evidence for the moderating effects of exercise participation. The type of exercise intervention was analysed amongst 6 eligible studies in the management of vasomotor menopausal symptoms and was compared to HRT. There was insufficient evidence demonstrating that exercise was effective in treating vasomotor menopausal symptoms, and, it was not clear whether exercise was more beneficial compared to HRT or yoga. In addition, data from the Australian Longitudinal Study on Women's Health including 3330 women suggested that no improvements in vasomotor or psychological symptoms and only marginal improvements in somatic symptoms were noted when physical activity was introduced as a factor influencing these symptoms. In a study of 280 women, increasing physical activity had no effect on vasomotor and sexual symptoms of menopause, and, in 24 women participating in a 3-month physical exercise protocol there were no improvements in sexual function. In a number of studies including, 16000 USA women, 173 African American and Caucasian women, and in 338 overweight women, no associations were found between physical activity and vasomotor symptoms. Recently, in a randomised controlled study of 237 women partaking in yoga classes, no improvement to vasomotor symptoms frequency were noted. Likewise, in 164 women partaking moderate physical activity, including walking and yoga, for 4 months, yielded no improvements in sleep quality in menopausal women. In another randomised controlled trial in 3 different sites, which involved 106 women to moderate exercise for 12 weeks and 142 women with no addition of exercise to their daily routine, did not improve vasomotor symptoms, however, small improvements were seen in sleep quality, insomnia and mood including depression. A cross sectional study of 1071 postmenopausal Turkish women who attended an outpatient clinic from 2005 to 2012, demonstrated no association between regular exercise and urogenital symptoms. Further, in a Norwegian study of 2002 women there was no relation amongst symptom burden and degree of physical exercise. Likewise, in a Nigerian population of 547 women there was no association with physical activity and menopausal symptoms and overall health related problems. These findings demonstrate that physical exercise has not consistently been shown to be beneficial in ameliorating symptoms associated to menopause.

Important reasons for the equivocal findings on the benefits of exercise on menopausal symptoms are the fact that studies have often assessed physical activity and exercise behaviours by means of self-report rather than objectively. In addition, exercise mode, intensity, frequency and duration has varied across the different studies making generalisations difficult. Finally, some studies have used participants who were already active prior to menopause whereas others include women who started exercise to alleviate symptoms. Different mechanisms might underlie symptomology in those are active prior to and during menopause versus those who take up exercise during menopause.

EXERCISE BEYOND MENOPAUSE

Habitual activity has numerous health benefits, including decreased risk or cardiorespiratory problems, metabolic syndromes, cancer and improved muscle and bone health and psychological symptoms. The risk of having one of these health issues is most prevalent postmenopause. Cardiovascular disease is increased in postmenopausal women, and the risk is lower in physically active women, by improving antioxidant capacity and decreasing body iron burden. Blood pressure is lower is physically active postmenopausal women compared to healthy sedentary women, and, resistance training with an intensity of 60% of 1 repeat for 12 weeks has beneficial effects on blood pressure, heart rate and cholesterol levels. Likewise, a modified relaxation technique intervention in Thai postmenopausal women had positive effects in lowering blood pressure as soon as 4 weeks after start of treatment. Interestingly, whole body vibration exercise training improves blood pressure, systemic and leg arterial stiffness, and muscle strength, in postmenopausal women although vibration exercise is not without risks. In addition, cardiorespiratory exercise improves metabolic syndrome effects (waist circumference, blood pressure and fasting glucose in postmenopausal women. Further, aerobic exercise and calorie restriction improves insulin sensitivity and reduces the risk of diabetes in postmenopausal women. Decrease in bone mineral density is associated with post menopause, and, walking for more than 6 months improves femoral neck bone mineral density in menopause women as analysed in 10 different trials. Further, skeletal muscle regeneration efficiency declines with age and is related to the decline in sex hormones. Long term resistance training increases muscle strength in postmenopausal women. Clinical trials are currently being undertaken to determine the effects of exercise on skeletal muscle regeneration and maintenance of muscle mass in postmenopausal women. Physical activity plays a pivotal role in maintaining health and prevent disease beyond menopause, including reduction in cardiovascular disease, breast cancer and diabetes, increasing muscle and bone mass, improving mood and cognitive functioning and overall quality of life. It is important for exercise to play a major role in postmenopausal women, to decrease the risks of disease and improve quality of life.

Tense about Exercise?

Physical activity during the menopause transition and post menopause, offers many benefits such as, weight gain prevention, strengthens bones and increases muscle mass and reduces the risks of other diseases (cancer, diabetes, heart disease). Exercise intervention programs have demonstrated to reduce menopause symptoms, including those of somatic, psychological and to a lesser extent vasomotor and sexual symptoms. Exercise has not been proven to treat menopausal symptoms, however, physically active women during and after menopause are less stressed and have better overall quality of life. Overall, the evidence suggests that exercise is a useful intervention strategy for women during and post menopause to alleviate symptoms. More importantly, exercise has numerous other benefits and is safe with no reported side-effects.

Future prospects

Due to inconsistencies associated with effects of exercise to menopause symptoms, in particular those relating to vasomotor symptoms, better designed and sufficiently powered randomised trials are required to understand the benefits of exercise and menopause symptoms. The inconsistencies reported may be due to varying sample sizes, non-randomised designs, inadequate specified exercise dose (vigorous vs moderate intensity; frequency, duration), mode (aerobic vs resistance exercise), and lack of follow-up. To this effect, a randomised control study over 12 months, is currently being conducted in 261 women to determine physical activity and its effects on hot flashes, night sweats and other menopausal symptoms. Further, the Menopause Strategies: Findings Lasting Awareness for Symptoms and Health (MeFLASH) Network, a collaborative project at 5 clinical sites in USA, is currently undertaking a 3 by 2 factorial design study assessing yoga, exercise and omega-3 supplementation and their effects on menopause symptoms. Interestingly in the MeFLASH trial, 112 previously sedentary women with hot flashes are randomised into moderate to vigorous exercise and are compared to 150 active control women. Findings will help aid in determining whether physical activity has any effects on menopause symptoms, in particular to vasomotor symptoms.

Previous research has shown that weight is associated to menopause symptoms. A study involving 3330 women in the Australian Longitudinal Study on Women's Health demonstrated a clear relationship with total and vasomotor symptoms and weight loss. In an 8 year follow up study of 1165 Finnish women, those whose weight remained stable improved their quality of life compared to women who had gained weight. Vasomotor symptoms such as hot flashes and night sweats are more prevalent in women with higher body mass index, and in an intensive behavioural weight loss intervention study, which included physical activity, in obese women, resulted in improvement in hot flashes. Conversely, 430 women in a 6-month controlled study demonstrated no associations of weight change with mental and physical quality of life. Future studies should involve weight or weight loss, by means of physical activity, and their effects on menopausal symptoms.

There are many known benefits of exercise on bone, cardiovascular, metabolic, and psychological health. Regular exercise is known to boost the immune system, and, decreases inflammation in menopausal women. Studies relating physical activity, to, immunological status, to, menopausal symptoms, during menopause and beyond, hold the key to understanding the underlying mechanisms to menopause symptoms.

4

High Intensity Training Interval

High Intensity Interval Training (HIIT) is a dynamic and time-efficient fitness approach that alternates short bursts of intense exercise with brief recovery periods. This method challenges the body to maximize calorie burn and improve cardiovascular fitness in a shorter timeframe compared to traditional workouts. HIIT's versatility accommodates various exercises, from sprinting to bodyweight routines, making it accessible to individuals with diverse fitness levels. With its proven ability to boost metabolism, enhance endurance, and promote fat loss, HIIT has gained widespread popularity as an effective and efficient workout strategy, revolutionizing the way people approach fitness for optimal results in minimal time.

Sprint interval training (SIT) is a form of high-intensity interval training (HIIT) that involves short bursts of intense exercise followed by periods of rest or lower-intensity activity. SIT has gained popularity for its efficiency in improving cardiovascular fitness, burning calories, and promoting overall health. Here's a breakdown of SIT:

TYPES OF SPRINT INTERNVAL TRAINING

Traditional SIT:

- Involves short, maximal effort sprints followed by brief rest periods.
- For example, 20-30 seconds of all-out sprinting followed by 30-60 seconds of rest or lower-intensity activity.

Tabata Protocol:

- Named after Dr. Izumi Tabata, it consists of 20 seconds of intense exercise followed by 10 seconds of rest, repeated for a total of 4 minutes.
- Common exercises include sprints, cycling, or bodyweight exercises.

30-Second Intervals:

- Similar to traditional SIT but with slightly longer sprint intervals.
- May involve 30 seconds of high-intensity exercise followed by 30-60 seconds of rest.

Hill Sprints:

- Performing sprints uphill adds an extra challenge and engages different muscle groups.
- Duration and intensity can vary based on fitness level and terrain.

Tips for Mastering Sprint Interval Training

Warm-up:

- Begin with a thorough warm-up to prepare your muscles and joints for the intense exercise.

Include dynamic stretches and a light cardiovascular activity.

Start Gradually:

- If you're new to SIT or have any health concerns, start with shorter intervals and lower intensity.

- Gradually increase the duration and intensity as your fitness improves.

Proper Form:

- Maintain proper form during sprints to reduce the risk of injury.
- Focus on good posture, arm movement, and controlled breathing.

Rest and Recovery:

- Allow adequate rest between sprint intervals to recover.
- Adequate recovery is crucial for preventing overtraining and reducing the risk of injuries.

Combine with Other Exercises:

- Include a variety of exercises in your SIT routine to target different muscle groups and prevent monotony.

Listen to Your Body:

- Pay attention to how your body responds to SIT.
- If you experience pain or discomfort, adjust the intensity or consult a fitness professional.

Stay Hydrated:

- Proper hydration is essential, especially during intense workouts.
- Drink water before, during, and after your SIT session.

BENEFITS OF SPRINT INTERVAL TRAINING FOR MENOPAUSAL WOMEN

Weight Management and Fat Loss

Menopausal hormonal changes can lead to weight gain and an increased risk of obesity. SIT has been shown to be effective in burning calories and promoting fat loss, making it a valuable tool for weight management during menopause.

Cardiovascular Health

Menopausal women often face an increased risk of cardiovascular issues. SIT helps improve cardiovascular health by enhancing heart function, reducing blood pressure, and increasing circulation.

Bone Health

Maintaining bone density is crucial for menopausal women, as the risk of osteoporosis increases. While SIT primarily focuses on cardiovascular fitness, its impact on overall health can indirectly contribute to bone health through weight-bearing exercises and improved hormonal balance.

Metabolic Health

SIT has been shown to enhance insulin sensitivity and glucose metabolism, which can be beneficial for managing metabolic issues that may arise during menopause, such as insulin resistance.

Hormonal Balance

Regular SIT can positively impact hormonal balance by promoting the release of endorphins, the body's natural mood enhancers. This can help alleviate symptoms such as mood swings and stress commonly associated with menopause.

Time Efficiency

Menopausal women often juggle multiple responsibilities, making time a precious commodity. SIT offers a time-efficient alternative to traditional, longer-duration workouts, as it can deliver significant health benefits in shorter sessions.

5

Strength Training in Menopause

As women athletes undergo the intricate transition of menopause, the intersection of strength training becomes a paramount consideration for sustaining peak performance and overall health. This chapter delves into the nuanced dynamics of strength training tailored specifically for women athletes navigating the challenges of menopause. Exploring the symbiotic relationship between hormonal changes and physical resilience, it examines how strategic strength training not only counters muscle loss and bone density decline but also enhances athletic prowess. Within this context, the chapter delineates personalized approaches, empowering women athletes to optimize their training regimens, foster resilience, and excel in their athletic pursuits amid the transformative journey of menopause.

THE IMPORTANCE OF HEAVY LIFTING

Incorporating heavy lifting can offer numerous benefits that contribute to overall health, well-being, and mitigating some of the challenges associated with this life stage. Here are several key reasons highlighting the importance of heavy lifting during menopause:

Preservation of Lean Muscle Mass

Menopause is often accompanied by hormonal changes, particularly a decline in estrogen levels. This hormonal shift can contribute to the loss of lean muscle mass. Heavy lifting, specifically resistance training with weights, helps to counteract this by stimulating the growth and maintenance of muscle tissue.

Bone Density Maintenance

Menopausal women are at an increased risk of osteoporosis due to a decrease in estrogen, which plays a role in bone density maintenance. Heavy lifting, especially weight-bearing exercises, imposes stress on the bones, promoting bone remodeling and strength. This can be crucial in preventing osteoporosis and reducing the risk of fractures.

Maintenance of Healthy Body Composition

Lifting heavy weights helps maintain lean muscle mass and reduces fat gain. As estrogen declines, the anabolic stimulus for muscle building diminishes, making it easier to accumulate fat, especially around the abdomen. Heavy resistance training signals the need for muscle strength, promoting lean mass development and decreasing central and total body fat.

Metabolic Boost

As people age, their metabolism tends to slow down. Heavy lifting, particularly compound exercises involving large muscle groups, can rev up the metabolism. This, in turn, helps with weight management and maintaining a healthy body composition, which is essential during menopause when weight gain is a common concern.

Hormonal Regulation

Strength training, especially with heavy loads, can positively impact hormonal balance. It can lead to the release of endorphins, the "feel-good" hormones, reducing stress and enhancing mood. Additionally, strength training has been associated with improved insulin sensitivity, which is important for managing blood sugar levels.

Enhanced Blood Pressure Control

Contrary to conventional wisdom, heavy lifting positively impacts cardiovascular health. It improves vascular compliance, aiding blood vessels in dilating and constricting more effectively. This results in better blood pressure control, improved blood flow to muscles, and enhanced circulation, crucial during menopause when cardiovascular disease risk rises.

Joint Health and Function

Menopausal women may experience changes in joint health, including a higher risk of arthritis. Heavy lifting, when done with proper form and technique, strengthens the muscles around joints, providing support and reducing the risk of joint-related issues.

Functional Strength for Daily Activities

Heavy lifting helps improve overall functional strength, making it easier for women to perform daily activities and maintain an active lifestyle. This is especially relevant during menopause when some women may experience a decline in energy levels and physical capabilities.

Increased Energy and Vitality

Engaging in heavy lifting can lead to increased energy levels and a sense of vitality. Regular strength training sessions have been linked to improved sleep quality, which is often disrupted during menopause. Better sleep contributes to overall well-being and helps manage symptoms such as mood swings and fatigue.

Empowerment and Confidence

Successfully lifting heavy weights can instill a sense of empowerment and confidence. This is particularly important during menopause, as some women may grapple with changes in body image and self-esteem. Achieving strength and fitness goals can positively impact mental and emotional well-being.

Improved Posture and Stability

Aging, coupled with menopause, can lead to joint issues. Heavy lifting stimulates tendons, enhancing their tension and overall joint stability. This effect extends to muscles indirectly involved, such as those supporting the spine, contributing to better posture and overall muscle health.

HOW TO EFFECTIVELY LIFT HEAVY AND ADDITIONAL TIPS

This guide aims to provide a comprehensive roadmap for incorporating heavy lifting into your fitness routine during menopause. We will explore the benefits of lifting heavy, the science behind its effectiveness, and practical steps to integrate this powerful practice into your daily life. Whether you are a novice or an experienced fitness enthusiast, the principles outlined here will empower you to embrace the potential of heavy lifting as a tool for vitality, resilience, and lasting health.

As we navigate the intricacies of menopause and strength training, remember that this is a personal journey one that can be adapted to suit your individual needs, preferences, and goals. Let's embark on this transformative path together, discovering the strength that lies within and harnessing the potential to thrive during the menopausal years.

Assess Current Fitness Level

Before starting any heavy lifting program, it's essential to assess your current fitness level. This can include evaluating your strength, flexibility, and any existing medical conditions. Consult with a healthcare professional or fitness expert to ensure that heavy lifting is appropriate for you.

Set Clear Goals

Define your specific goals for strength training during menopause. Whether it's improving muscle mass, bone density, overall strength, or addressing specific health concerns, having clear objectives will help tailor your program to your needs.

Learn Proper Technique

Proper technique is crucial for heavy lifting to ensure safety and effectiveness. Work with a certified personal trainer or strength coach to learn the correct form for exercises like squats, deadlifts, bench presses, and overhead presses. This will minimize the risk of injury and maximize the benefits of your training.

Start with a Warm-up

Warm up your muscles and joints with 10-15 minutes of light aerobic exercise, such as brisk walking or cycling. Follow this with dynamic stretching to prepare your body for the upcoming heavy lifting session.

Follow A Mobility Session

Prioritize a 10 to 15-minute warm-up, incorporating foam rolling and mobility exercises. The strength trainers with extensive experience, recommends the following routine:

Twist Hip Opener: Kneel, holding a light weight, rotate while pressing hips forward. Repeat for 10 reps. Switch sides.

Open Hip Toggle: Kneel and sway hips side to side while holding a foam roller overhead. Repeat for 10 reps on each side. Switch sides.

Foam Roll Lower Leg: Sit on the floor with legs straight, supporting weight on hands. Roll the calf from ankle to knee for 30 seconds. Switch legs.

T Spine Extension: Lie back on a foam roller, extending back and curling forward for 60 seconds to massage the upper back.

Dowel Hip Opener: Kneel, holding a dowel overhead, and pressing hips forward and back. Repeat for 10 repetitions. Switch sides.

Foam Roll Posterior Hip: Cross right ankle over left knee, rolling glutes back and forth over the roller for 30 seconds. Switch sides.

Progressive Overload

To build strength, gradually increase the amount of weight you lift over time. This is known as progressive overload. Start with a weight that challenges you but allows for proper form. As you get stronger, gradually increase the resistance.

Choose Compound Exercises

Compound exercises involve multiple muscle groups and joints, making them efficient for building overall strength. Examples include squats, deadlifts, bench presses, and overhead presses. Incorporate these into your routine for a well-rounded approach.

Plan Your Workout

Structure your workouts to target different muscle groups on different days. For example, you might have a day dedicated to lower body exercises (e.g., squats and lunges) and another day for upper body exercises (e.g., bench presses and rows). This allows for adequate rest between muscle groups.

Include Recovery Days

Recovery is crucial, especially during menopause when hormonal changes may affect recovery rates. Ensure you have rest days between heavy lifting sessions to allow your muscles to recover and adapt.

Listen to Your Body

Pay attention to how your body responds to heavy lifting. If you experience pain (other than normal muscle soreness), fatigue, or any unusual discomfort, it's important to address it. Consult with a healthcare professional or adjust your training program accordingly.

HYDRATION THROUGH EXERCISE AND BEYOND

Water Intake

Aim for at least 8-10 glasses (64-80 ounces) of water per day. This can vary based on individual factors like body weight, activity level, and climate.

Carry a reusable water bottle to make it easy to track and maintain hydration throughout the day.

Drink water before, during, and after strength training sessions.

Electrolyte Balance

Electrolytes play a crucial role in hydration. Ensure an adequate intake of potassium, sodium, calcium, and magnesium.

Include potassium-rich foods like bananas, oranges, and leafy greens in your diet.

Use electrolyte supplements or sports drinks during intense workouts, particularly if you're sweating heavily.

Pre-Workout Hydration

Consume water before starting your strength training session. Aim to drink around 16-20 ounces of water 2-3 hours before exercising.

Drink an additional 8-10 ounces about 20-30 minutes before your workout.

Hydration during Exercise

Sip water throughout your strength training session to maintain hydration levels.

Consider the intensity and duration of your workout when determining how much water to drink during exercise.

Post-Workout Rehydration

Rehydrate after your workout to replace fluids lost through sweat.

Drink at least 16-24 ounces of water within two hours of finishing your strength training session.

Monitor Urine Color

Use the color of your urine as a simple indicator of hydration. Pale yellow to light straw color generally indicates good hydration.

Limit Caffeine and Alcohol

Both caffeine and alcohol can contribute to dehydration. Limit their intake and balance with increased water consumption.

Include Hydrating Foods

Incorporate water-rich foods into your diet, such as fruits (watermelon, cucumber, berries) and vegetables (lettuce, celery, and tomatoes).

Listen to Your Body

Pay attention to thirst signals. If you feel thirsty, it's a sign that your body needs more fluids.

Adapt to Menopausal Symptoms

Hot flashes and night sweats can contribute to fluid loss. Adjust your hydration strategy accordingly during and after these episodes.

OTHER ESSENTIAL HEAVY LIFTING EXERCISES

Squats and Their Types

1. Bodyweight Squat:

- Description: The basic squat involves standing with feet shoulder-width apart and lowering your body as if you were sitting back into a chair.
- Benefits: Builds strength in the lower body, engages core muscles, and improves mobility.
- Duration: Beginners may start with 2-3 sets of 10-15 reps, gradually increasing as strength improves.

2. Goblet Squat:

- Description: Hold a dumbbell or kettlebell close to your chest as you perform the squat.
- Benefits: Adds resistance to the squat, engaging the upper body and core in addition to the lower body.
- Duration: 3-4 sets of 8-12 reps.

3. Front Squat:

- Description: Barbell is placed across the front of the shoulders instead of the back.
- Benefits: Emphasizes the quadriceps and core, encourages an upright posture.
- Duration: 3-4 sets of 6-10 reps.

4. Back Squat:

- Description: Barbell is placed across the upper back.
- Benefits: Targets the posterior chain, including hamstrings and glutes.
- Duration: 3-4 sets of 6-10 reps.

5. Overhead Squat:

- Description: Squat while holding a weight overhead.
- Benefits: Requires excellent mobility and engages the entire body.
- Duration: 3 sets of 8-12 reps.

6. Split Squat:

- Description: Stand with one foot forward and the other back, lowering your body into a lunge position.
- Benefits: Works each leg individually, improving balance and addressing muscle imbalances.
- Duration: 3 sets of 8-12 reps per leg.

Duration and Frequency:

- Frequency: Aim for 2-3 strength training sessions per week, allowing at least one day of rest between sessions.
- Duration: The duration of a squat workout can vary. A well-rounded strength training session may take 45-60 minutes, including warm-up and cool-down. The duration of each squat exercise should be tailored to individual fitness levels, with an emphasis on proper form.

Deadlift

The deadlift stands as a symbol of raw strength and resilience, demanding both physical prowess and mental fortitude. This compound movement engages multiple muscle groups simultaneously, making it a powerhouse exercise for overall strength development. As women enter menopause, maintaining and even enhancing physical strength becomes pivotal for their well-being, both in terms of managing hormonal changes and optimizing overall health.

The deadlift, in its various forms and variations, is a foundational exercise that has stood the test of time. It epitomizes functional strength, mimicking the everyday movement of picking objects up from the ground. This primal action becomes increasingly significant as women in menopause strive to preserve their independence, agility, and vitality.

Conventional Deadlift

The traditional deadlift form involves a hip-width stance with the hands gripping the bar just outside the knees. This classic variation targets the posterior chain, including the hamstrings, glutes, lower back, and traps.

Sumo Deadlift

Widening the stance and positioning the hands inside the knees characterizes the sumo deadlift. This variation places more emphasis on the inner thighs and quads, providing a unique challenge to different muscle groups.

Romanian Deadlift (RDL)

The Romanian deadlift focuses on the eccentric phase of the lift, emphasizing the stretch and contraction of the hamstrings and lower back. It's an excellent variation for building muscle endurance and promoting flexibility.

Trap Bar Deadlift

Utilizing a trap bar alters the mechanics of the deadlift, offering a more upright posture and reducing stress on the lower back. This variation is particularly beneficial for those with lower back concerns.

CROSSFIT FITNESS EXERCISES

Designing a CrossFit fitness routine for menopausal women involves a balanced approach that addresses both the unique challenges and advantages associated with this life stage. Before beginning any new fitness program, it's crucial to consult with a healthcare professional and a qualified fitness trainer to ensure it aligns with individual health considerations. Here's a sample CrossFit-inspired routine tailored for menopausal women:

Warm-Up (5-10 minutes)

- Jumping jacks: 2 minutes
- Arm circles: 1 minute
- High knees: 2 minutes
- Dynamic stretching (leg swings, hip circles): 3 minutes
- Light jogging in place: 2 minutes

- Workout: CrossFit Circuit (Repeat for 3 Rounds)

1. Box Jumps

- 15 reps
- Use a sturdy box or step.
- Focus on controlled movements to engage lower body muscles.

2. Kettlebell Swings

- 20 reps
- Use a moderate-weight kettlebell.
- Engage the hips and core for a powerful swing motion.

3. Push-Ups

- 12 reps
- Modify as needed (on knees or against a raised surface).
- Focus on maintaining a straight line from head to heels.

4. Dumbbell Rows

- 12 reps per arm
- Use moderate-weight dumbbells.
- Maintain a stable core and controlled movement.

5. Double-Unders or Single-Unders (Jump Rope)

- 2 minutes
- Adjust intensity based on individual fitness level.
- Improve cardiovascular health and coordination.

6. Plank Hold

- 1 minute

- Engage the core and maintain a straight line from head to heels.
- Modify by dropping to forearms if needed.

Cool Down (5-10 minutes)

- Foam rolling: Focus on major muscle groups, especially legs and back.
- Static stretching: Hold each stretch for 15-30 seconds for major muscle groups (hamstrings, quadriceps, chest, shoulders).
- Deep breathing exercises: 5 minutes to promote relaxation and recovery.

MAINTAINING BRACED NEUTRAL SPINE

Maintaining a properly braced neutral spine is crucial during exercise, especially for women going through menopause. A neutral spine refers to the natural, S-shaped curvature of your spine when it is in a balanced and aligned position. This position helps distribute forces evenly, reducing the risk of injury and promoting optimal movement patterns. Here's a detailed guide on how to maintain a properly braced neutral spine during various exercises:

Understanding Neutral Spine

- The natural curves of the spine include the cervical (neck), thoracic (mid-back), and lumbar (lower back) regions.

- A neutral spine preserves these curves, avoiding excessive flexion (forward bending) or extension (backward arching).
- Engaging the core muscles plays a crucial role in supporting a neutral spine.

Core Engagement

- **Pelvic Floor Activation:** Initiate by engaging the pelvic floor muscles, as if you are stopping the flow of urine.
- **Transverse Abdominis (TA) Activation:** Imagine tightening your abdominal muscles, pulling your belly button towards your spine.
- **Maintain Engagement:** Keep the core muscles activated throughout the exercise to provide stability to the spine.

Proper Body Alignment

- **Head and Neck:** Maintain a neutral position by aligning your head with your spine. Avoid looking up or down excessively.
- **Shoulders:** Keep the shoulders relaxed and avoid rounding or hunching forward.
- **Hips:** Align your hips with your spine. Avoid tilting the pelvis excessively forward or backward.

Breathing Technique

- **Inhale:** Take a deep breath before initiating the movement.

- **Exhale:** Exhale during the effort phase of the exercise. This helps maintain intra-abdominal pressure and supports the spine.

Start with Bodyweight Exercises

- Begin with exercises that use your body weight before progressing to weighted exercises.
- Focus on form and gradually increase intensity.

Consultation with a Professional

- If possible, seek guidance from a fitness professional or physical therapist to ensure proper form and technique.

Regular Monitoring

- Pay attention to your body and how it feels during and after exercises. Adjust your form if you experience discomfort.

Flexibility and Mobility

- Include stretching and mobility exercises to maintain flexibility, which can contribute to better spinal alignment.

Adapt to Individual Needs

- Recognize that everyone's body is different. Adapt exercises based on individual flexibility, strength, and any pre-existing conditions.

6

Let's Start Jumping Through Menopause

Plyometrics, also known as jump training or shock training, involves rapid contraction and extension of muscles, with the aim of increasing power and strength. While plyometrics is often associated with athletes, it can also offer numerous benefits for older women, particularly those going through menopause.

BENEFITS OF PLYOMETRICS

Bone Density Improvement

Menopause is associated with a decline in estrogen levels, which can lead to a decrease in bone density. Plyometric exercises, especially weight-bearing ones, can help improve bone density. The impact and loading on bones during plyometrics stimulate bone formation, contributing to increased bone density and reducing the risk of osteoporosis.

Muscle Strength and Power

Plyometrics involve explosive movements that engage various muscle groups. For women in menopause, maintaining muscle strength becomes crucial, as muscle mass tends to decrease with age. Improved muscle strength and power can enhance daily activities, reduce the risk of falls, and contribute to overall functional fitness.

Joint Health

Menopausal women often experience joint pain and stiffness due to hormonal changes. Plyometric exercises can help maintain joint health by promoting flexibility and strengthening the muscles around the joints. This can alleviate discomfort and improve overall joint function.

Metabolic Boost

As metabolism tends to slow down with age, maintaining a healthy weight becomes challenging. Plyometric exercises, being high-intensity and metabolically demanding, can contribute to weight management and fat loss. This is essential for women in menopause as hormonal changes may lead to weight gain, especially around the abdomen.

Improved Cardiovascular Health

Plyometric exercises can elevate the heart rate, contributing to cardiovascular health. Engaging in these activities may help manage cardiovascular risk factors that become more prominent during menopause, such as increased cholesterol levels and reduced cardiovascular fitness.

Mood and Cognitive Benefits

Regular physical activity, including plyometrics, has been linked to improved mood and cognitive function. Menopause can bring about mood swings and cognitive changes, and incorporating plyometrics into a fitness routine may help alleviate these symptoms by promoting the release of endorphins and supporting brain health.

Enhanced Balance and Coordination

Plyometrics require coordinated movements and balance, which can be beneficial for older women. Improving balance and coordination is crucial for preventing falls, which become a significant concern during menopause due to changes in bone density and muscle mass.

Social and Psychological Well-being

Engaging in plyometric exercises in a group setting or with a workout partner can provide social interaction and emotional support. This can positively impact mental health, reducing feelings of isolation and promoting a sense of well-being.

LET'S START WITH JUMP TRANING

Similar to potent medicine, a minimal amount of plyometrics yields substantial benefits. Just 10 minutes, three times weekly, is sufficient for jumping exercises. Gradual introduction is crucial to ensure connective tissues are conditioned for impact.

Low-Impact Plyometrics

- Description: Perform exercises with reduced impact to protect joints.
- Examples: Low-impact squat jumps, step-ups, and lateral leg raises.

Box Jumps

- Description: Jumping onto and off of a sturdy box to enhance lower body power.
- Modification: Start with a lower box height and gradually increase as strength improves.

Jump Rope

- Description: Incorporate skipping or jumping rope for cardiovascular conditioning and lower body strength.
- Modification: Begin with slow, controlled jumps and progress to higher intensity as fitness levels improve.

Bounding

- Description: Perform long, exaggerated strides emphasizing power and coordination.
- Modification: Keep bounding movements controlled and focus on proper landing mechanics.

Medicine Ball Throws

- Description: Explosive movements involving throwing and catching a medicine ball.
- Modification: Start with a lighter medicine ball and gradually progress to heavier ones as strength increases.

Single-Leg Jumps

- Description: Focus on one leg at a time to improve balance and stability.
- Modification: Begin with small jumps and progress to higher intensity while maintaining proper form.

Agility Drills

- Description: Incorporate ladder drills, cone drills, and other agility exercises for improved coordination.

- Modification: Perform exercises at a pace that allows for control and accuracy.

Pool Plyometrics

- Description: Conduct jump training in water to reduce impact on joints.
- Modification: Adjust the intensity by controlling the depth of water and the speed of movements.

Resistance Band Jumps:

- Description: Use resistance bands to add resistance to jumping movements, targeting muscles more effectively.
- Modification: Start with lighter resistance and progress as strength improves.

Bodyweight Exercises

- Description: Utilize bodyweight exercises like squat jumps, burpees, and tuck jumps.
- Modification: Perform controlled movements to minimize impact on joints.

Squat Jump

- Stand with feet wider than shoulder-width apart, arms extended in front. Squat down, then explosively jump, landing softly and immediately repeating 8 to 10 times. Begin with one set and progress to two, either in the morning and evening or consecutively.
- Once comfortable, advance to circuit training, performing various jump exercises consecutively, with a suggested 45

seconds "on" (jumping) and 15 seconds "off" (resting) for three circuits. Beginners start with one circuit, gradually increasing.

Mountain Climber

- Start in a high plank and drive knees toward the chest in a running motion, maintaining a straight line from head to heels.

7

Understanding Menopause and Core Strength

Hormonal changes during this period, especially a decline in estrogen levels, can contribute to several physical changes, including a decrease in muscle mass and bone density. These changes can impact core strength, leading to issues such as weakened abdominal muscles, reduced pelvic floor support, and an increased risk of lower back pain.

CHALLENGES FACED TO MAINTAIN CORE STRENGTH

Muscle Loss

Estrogen plays a crucial role in maintaining muscle mass. As estrogen levels decline during menopause, women may experience a gradual loss of muscle, including the muscles that make up the core.

Bone Density Reduction

The decline in estrogen also affects bone density, making women more susceptible to conditions like osteoporosis. Weakened bones can compromise the stability of the spine and negatively impact core strength.

Hormonal Fluctuations

Hormonal fluctuations during menopause can lead to weight gain, particularly around the abdominal area. Excess weight can place additional stress on the core muscles, making it challenging to maintain strength.

TIPS FOR MAINTAINING CORE STRENGTH

Regular Exercise: Engage in a combination of aerobic exercises, strength training, and flexibility exercises. Cardiovascular activities, such as brisk walking, swimming, or cycling, help maintain overall fitness.

Incorporate strength training exercises targeting the core muscles, including the abdominals, obliques, and lower back.

Specific Core Exercises: Planks, bridges, and pelvic tilts are excellent exercises for targeting the core. These exercises help strengthen the abdominal muscles, lower back, and pelvic floor.

Yoga and Pilates are also effective for enhancing core strength while promoting flexibility and balance.

Balanced Diet: Ensure a diet rich in calcium and vitamin D to support bone health. Include dairy products, leafy greens, and fortified foods in your meals.

Adequate protein intake is essential for muscle maintenance and repair. Include lean protein sources such as poultry, fish, beans, and nuts.

Posture Awareness: Maintain good posture throughout the day to reduce strain on the back and core muscles. Sit and stand tall, and be mindful of your body alignment.

Stress Management: Chronic stress can contribute to weight gain and muscle tension. Incorporate stress-reducing activities such as meditation, deep breathing, or mindfulness practices.

Consultation with Healthcare Professionals: Regular check-ups with healthcare providers can help monitor bone density and address any emerging health concerns. Discuss any changes in your exercise routine or symptoms with your healthcare team.

CORE STRENGTHENING EXERCISES

Core strengthening exercises focus on improving the strength and stability of the core or canister which includes the muscles of the abdomen, lower back, hips, and pelvic floor. A strong and stable core is crucial for maintaining proper posture, preventing injuries, and supporting various daily activities. Here are detailed exercises to strengthen the core:

Pelvic Tilts

- Lie on your back with knees bent and feet flat on the floor.
- Inhale and engage your pelvic floor muscles.
- Exhale and tilt your pelvis upward, pressing your lower back into the floor.
- Hold for a moment, then release. Repeat for 10-15 repetitions.

Bridge Exercise

- Lie on your back with knees bent and feet hip-width apart.
- Inhale and engage your core muscles.

- Exhale as you lift your hips towards the ceiling, creating a straight line from shoulders to knees.
- Hold at the top for a moment, then lower back down. Repeat for 12-15 repetitions.

Plank Variations

- **Standard Plank:** Begin in a plank position with wrists directly under shoulders. Hold for 20-30 seconds, gradually increasing over time.
- **Side Plank:** Rotate into a side plank, balancing on one forearm with the body in a straight line. Hold for 15-20 seconds on each side.

Dead Bug Exercise

- Lie on your back with arms extended towards the ceiling and legs lifted off the ground.
- Lower the right arm and left leg towards the floor simultaneously, keeping the lower back pressed into the ground.
- Return to the starting position and switch sides. Repeat for 12-15 repetitions on each side.

Bird Dog Exercise

- Start on your hands and knees in a table top position.
- Extend your right arm forward and left leg backward, keeping the spine neutral.
- Hold for a moment, then return to the starting position. Switch sides and repeat for 12-15 repetitions on each side.

Russian Twists

- Sit on the floor with knees bent and feet flat on the ground.
- Lean back slightly and lift your feet off the ground, balancing on your sit bones.
- Rotate your torso to the right, bringing your hands towards the floor beside you. Return to the center and then twist to the left. Repeat for 15-20 repetitions.

Superman Exercise

- Lie on your stomach with arms extended in front of you.
- Lift your arms, chest, and legs off the ground simultaneously, squeezing your glutes and lower back muscles.
- Hold for a moment, then lower back down. Repeat for 12-15 repetitions.

Seated Leg Lifts

- Sit on the edge of a chair with a straight back.
- Lift one leg straight out in front of you, engaging the core.
- Hold for a moment, then lower the leg back down. Repeat for 12-15 repetitions on each leg.

Cobra Stretch

- Lie on your stomach and place your hands under your shoulders.
- Inhale as you lift your chest off the ground, keeping your pelvis on the floor.

- Hold for a moment, then lower back down. Repeat for 12-15 repetitions.

Pelvic Floor Exercises (Kegels)

- Contract the pelvic floor muscles as if stopping the flow of urine.
- Hold for a few seconds, then release.
- Repeat for 10-15 repetitions, gradually increasing the duration of the holds.

8

Healthy Diet in Menopause

A Crucial element in optimizing health throughout the menopause journey is maintaining a healthy diet. Unfortunately, less than 20% of women in the United States adhere to a healthy diet during and after menopause. This is particularly disheartening considering the numerous benefits associated with a healthy diet, including reducing the risk of heart disease (the leading cause of death for women), minimizing the risk of type 2 diabetes, preventing constipation and hemorrhoids, lowering the risk of colon cancer, and decreasing the risk of Alzheimer's disease.

Before delving into the topic, let's debunk the misattributed quote to Hippocrates: "Let food be thy medicine." Despite its widespread presence, this quote is a fabrication and doesn't appear in the extensive collection of works attributed to Hippocrates and his peers. This misinformation is prevalent in various sources, from medical journals to Instagram accounts advocating diets, even making its way into a post on Gwyneth Paltrow's goop.com. The importance of fact-checking in such contexts becomes evident.

The ancient Greeks made a clear distinction between food and medicine, recommending diets based on symptoms, sex, and season, although not necessarily grounded in scientific understanding. Their dietary practices were shaped by misconceptions about the human body and diseases, some of which modern science has debunked. Relying on ancient wisdom, especially when coupled with the natural fallacy (believing nature is inherently superior), complicates the already challenging task of distinguishing between food facts and fiction.

While certain foods can address specific deficiencies, such as oranges curing scurvy or red meat reversing iron deficiency, these instances involve treating dietary inadequacies rather than underlying medical conditions. Emphasizing a healthy diet as a form of preventative care is a medical truth often overlooked in discussions, overshadowed by interventions like menopausal hormone therapy (MHT) or supplements.

Several factors contribute to the neglect of diet discussions, including the limited time available in brief medical appointments, insufficient nutrition training for healthcare providers, and challenges in accessing qualified nutrition experts. Additionally, societal and medical fat phobia further sidelines the foundational benefits of a healthy diet, with messaging often focusing on perceived body issues rather than overall well-being.

When faced with unhelpful or dismissive responses from the medical community, individuals often seek alternative sources of information. This opens the door to nutrition charlatans, ranging from doctors and registered dietitians to influencers, making extravagant claims about the healing properties of trendy superfoods or offering bold promises of hormone resets. These purported solutions often come with a hefty price tag in the form of programs, supplements, or special teas.

FOOD SCIENCE AND ITS CHALLENGES

Communication and access challenges in nutrition aside, food science poses its own difficulties. Similar to how Big Pharma can influence medication studies through funding, biases can infiltrate nutrition studies. Moreover, the sheer volume of data generated often presents contradictions, making it challenging to discern dietary guidelines. The frequent shifts in consensus on whether certain foods are beneficial or harmful add to the confusion, akin to changing hemlines.

Studying diets is exceptionally complex. Observational studies, which identify dietary patterns linked to health outcomes, provide interesting insights but only establish associations. For instance, a lower incidence of hot flushes in East Asian women might be linked to higher soy consumption, but the causation is unclear. Various factors, such as lifelong soy consumption, dietary composition, genetics, or social determinants of health, could influence the observed association. Sometimes, associations may even be spurious, reflecting statistical anomalies rather than real connections.

Understanding how our bodies process food involves intricate complexities beyond single ingredients. While observational studies may inspire hypotheses, they rarely offer clean data for definitive conclusions. Intervention studies, where diets are randomly assigned and closely controlled, offer more comprehensive insights but are expensive and challenging to execute, as seen in the Women's

Health Initiative (WHI). The WHI's low-fat diet arm, intended to prevent breast cancer and other diseases, showed limited adherence and inconclusive results, emphasizing the challenges in implementing and interpreting dietary interventions.

To overcome the limitations of studying diets in real-life settings, some research facilities conduct studies with participants living on-site, where all food is prepared and tracked. However, these studies are short-term due to practical and financial constraints, and conflicting results may arise, as seen in comparing high-fat ketogenic and high-carbohydrate vegetarian diets. Despite these challenges, the evolving nature of scientific inquiry often raises more questions than answers. The desire for clear-cut dietary answers, shared by many, including doctors, has led to the allure of so-called superfoods. The rapid succession of superfoods, from apples to açai berries, turmeric, quinoa, kale, oatmeal, pomegranate, coconut oil, and celery juice, exemplifies the evolving and sometimes fickle nature of dietary trends.

NUTRITION 101

Macronutrients, such as protein (4 calories per gram), carbohydrates (4 calories per gram), and fat (9 calories per gram), serve as both energy sources and essential building blocks. For instance, protein's amino acids contribute to the creation of various structures, from enzymes to eyelashes, and fat's cholesterol is repurposed for functions ranging from cell membranes to estrogen synthesis.

Micronutrients, encompassing vital vitamins and minerals, are crucial for bodily functions and are required in small quantities, hence the term "micro." Examples include iron, iodine, folate, zinc, and vitamins A and C.

Carbohydrates, composed of sugar molecules, are categorized into simple and complex types. Simple carbohydrates, with one or two sugar molecules, are smaller and easier to digest. Examples include sugars like sucrose and glucose in fruits and vegetables, as well as galactose, lactose, table sugar, and high fructose corn syrup. Complex carbohydrates, consisting of three or more sugar molecules, encompass starches and fiber, with only starches being digestible. Starches are found in vegetables, legumes, nuts, and whole grains like oatmeal, whole wheat, brown rice, and quinoa. Refined grains, such as white flour and white rice, are simple carbohydrates lacking fiber and nutrients.

Both simple carbohydrates and starches break down into glucose, utilized immediately for energy, converted into glycogen, or repackaged and stored as fat. Simple carbohydrates are quickly digested, causing a rapid glucose influx into the bloodstream, while complex carbohydrates release glucose at a slower rate. Diets high in simple carbohydrates are associated with elevated risks of cardiovascular disease and type 2 diabetes.

A diet rich in refined carbohydrates is linked to lower sex hormone binding globulin (SHBG) levels, resulting in increased active estrogen and testosterone levels. This association may negatively impact hormonally responsive cancers, such as breast and endometrial cancers.

FIBER FOR A HEALTHIER, VIBRANT LIFE

Unlike many dietary interventions, it doesn't involve removing foods but rather focuses on adding something beneficial. Fiber, a nondigestible carbohydrate, comes in two types: soluble (dissolvable in water) and insoluble. Both types, often present together in the same food, offer health advantages. Women should aim for 25g of fiber daily, while men require 38g. Despite these recommendations, the average fiber intake in the United States is only 17g per day, with only 5 percent meeting the daily target.

Increasing fiber intake provides various health benefits, including enhanced fullness after meals due to increased bulk, stimulation of bowel activity reducing constipation, and a lowered risk of hemorrhoids. Fiber also slows carbohydrate digestion, reducing blood sugar spikes, and aids in cholesterol reduction, with postmenopausal women experiencing a greater response to fiber intake. Furthermore, fiber's impact on estrogen levels for premenopausal women may contribute to a lower risk of hormonally responsive breast cancers.

Fiber lowers stool pH, possesses anti-inflammatory properties, inhibits harmful bacteria growth, and boosts mineral absorption. Some soluble fiber acts as a prebiotic, encouraging the growth of healthy gut bacteria. Despite its many benefits, a high-fiber diet may result in gas, as seen with certain foods like Jerusalem artichokes.

A diet rich in fiber is linked to lower rates of cardiovascular disease, type 2 diabetes, and colon cancer. While fiber may aid in weight maintenance, this aspect is discussed only when patients inquire, as the focus is on the overall health benefits of fiber. Found in whole grains, legumes, fruits, and vegetables, fiber-rich foods also provide essential micronutrients. Wheat bran is particularly effective at bulking stool.

Encouraging women to track their food intake and adjust fiber accordingly is a straightforward dietary change. Adding high-fiber cereal or switching from white rice to brown rice are simple adjustments. Personally, I recommend high-fiber cereals such as Kashi Go Rise, Kellogg's All Bran, and Post Foods Uncle Sam for their nutritional content and palatability. The goal is not just having enough fiber but ensuring it's palatable enough for regular consumption.

PROCESSING OF FOOD

Natural food remains unchanged from its original form in nature examples include bananas, chickpeas, chicken, or honey. Any alteration to the fundamental nature of food, such as freezing, pasteurization, or sugar addition, is considered processing. Items like flour, cheese, tofu, and canned kidney beans undergo processing, including the surprising revelation that baby carrots are simply whittled-down versions of larger carrots.

While processed foods are often part of a nutritious diet and contribute to food safety and shelf life, the real concern lies with ultra-processed foods. These are typically industrial formulations with ingredients beyond salt, sugar, and fats not commonly used in home cooking. Ultra-processed foods constitute 58 percent of dietary energy consumed in America and contribute to 90 percent of added sugar intake.

Exceptions and confusion arise, as some packaged breakfast cereals are ultra-processed, yet some provide whole grains, fiber, and added micronutrients with minimal added sugar. Similarly, certain store-bought potato chips may consist of only potatoes, salt, and oil, but are still considered ultra-processed due to the lack of equipment for home production.

Ultra-processed foods, except for some cereals, are generally nutritionally incomplete, lacking essential micronutrients, and often lead to increased calorie consumption. Studies show that individuals on a diet of ultra-processed foods eat 500 more calories a day. Various factors contribute to this, including ease of chewing, less fiber leading to reduced fullness, significant fluctuations in glucose and insulin levels, and the irresistible taste of added sugar, fat, and salt.

These foods are linked to health issues such as abdominal obesity, metabolic syndrome, type 2 diabetes, hypertension, and cardiovascular disease. Given the prevalence of these conditions during menopause, eliminating ultra-processed foods becomes a crucial dietary recommendation after maximizing fiber intake. However, it's essential to acknowledge the privilege associated with eliminating ultra-processed foods, as social determinants of health and structural racism can limit access to fresh foods, and financial constraints and time limitations may hinder the adoption of healthier eating habits.

DIETARY FATS

Dietary fats fall into two categories: saturated and unsaturated, depending on the carbon-hydrogen bonding. Saturated fats, solid at room temperature, are derived from animal products like meat, dairy, and poultry. Unsaturated fats, found in fish, vegetables, nuts, and grains, can be monounsaturated or polyunsaturated, commonly known as omega-3 and omega-6 fatty acids.

While dietary fats play a crucial role in providing calories, aiding vitamin absorption, and serving as essential building blocks, excess fat is stored in adipose cells, convertible to glucose through ketogenesis. Low-fat diets lack proven health benefits, but the type of fat matters. Evidence indicates that a diet high in saturated fats is linked to an increased risk of cardiovascular disease and elevated LDL (bad cholesterol) levels. Conversely, unsaturated fats, prevalent in vegetable oils, nuts, and fish, have positive effects. Trans fats, produced industrially, are universally harmful and are now regulated out of food in the United States.

Omega-3 fatty acids, including ALA, EPA, and DHA, are noteworthy. ALA is found in flaxseed, walnuts, soybeans, canola oils, and omega-3 enriched eggs, while DHA and EPA are exclusive to fish and seafood. Omega-3s lower triglycerides, reduce atherosclerosis, and may decrease blood pressure, often requiring supplementation for postmenopausal women.

Linoleic acid, the primary omega-6 fatty acid in vegetable oils like corn, safflower, and flax seeds, lowers the risk of diabetes and promotes heart health. Balancing efforts to increase omega-3 fatty acids should not compromise omega-6 fatty acids, as both play essential roles.

CAFFEINE

It's mostly positive, well, almost entirely. Maybe you don't share my love for caffeine, but I'll admit my bias up front as a devoted enthusiast. I'm not alone 85 percent of U.S. adults consume caffeine daily, with coffee and tea ranking among the most globally popular beverages. Caffeine is also present in chocolate, sports drinks, and various plants and berries.

The overall data is reassuring up to five cups of coffee a day seems harmless and is linked to a reduced risk of mortality, liver and gallbladder diseases, and Parkinson's disease.

Caffeine may also lower the risk of depression, alleviate headaches, and enhance alertness. While some may experience negative effects on sleep and increased anxiety, caffeine poisoning is unlikely through regular food and drink consumption (requiring an excessive 75 to 100 cups). However, caution is advised with caffeine supplements.

A coffee-related caveat exists cafestol, a coffee chemical, can elevate cholesterol. Unfiltered coffee, like French press, contains the highest cafestol levels, followed by espresso, while drip and instant coffee have the lowest. Consuming over six cups a day of unfiltered coffee or espresso is associated with higher LDL cholesterol levels. Therefore, women with elevated LDL who enjoy unfiltered coffee or espresso might consider switching to drip. Personally, I stick to "four to five cups of espresso a day."

ALCOHOL

Alcohol has widespread effects on various organ systems, influencing sleep, hot flushes, libido, the brain, bones covered in relevant chapters. From an overall health perspective, alcohol and its toxic metabolites can harm the liver, heart, bones, and stomach. It also plays a role in accidents and homicides. Alcohol use is associated with several cancers, including breast, esophageal, and liver.

Alcohol might increase the risk of breast cancer through carcinogenic metabolites, its link with obesity, interference with estrogen metabolism in the liver, and impact on the production of SHBG (sex hormone binding globulin). In contrast, data suggests that low levels of alcohol intake, particularly red wine, may reduce the risk of heart attack. This duality showcases how a single food does not define a diet; alcohol may offer benefits in some contexts and amounts while posing risks in others.

For a healthy woman without alcoholism or liver disease, and who won't drink and drive, consuming less than 17 g of alcohol per day may yield some health benefits. In the United States, 12 ounces of regular beer (5 percent alcohol), 5 ounces of wine (12 percent alcohol), and 1.5 ounces of distilled spirit (40 percent alcohol) equal 14 g, or 1.75 units. These seven to nine drinks a week should be spread over at least three days, not concentrated in one night.

EATING PLANS AND MENOPAUSE

With these fundamental nutritional guidelines, what are the most effective dietary approaches for the menopause continuum?

The optimal diet for menopause generally prioritizes heart health, considering it is the leading cause of death in women. Ideally, this diet should also address the prevention of osteoporosis, Alzheimer's disease, and breast and endometrial cancer.

It's tempting to selectively use data to present a compelling argument for the superiority of one diet over another. However, many diets have both advantages and disadvantages, and the complexities of food science often lead to uncertainties and context-dependent outcomes. For instance, while it's recommended to limit saturated fats to less than 10 percent of daily calories (5-6 percent for a heart-healthy diet), an individual who achieves and maintains a 25 kg weight loss through a high-animal-fat, low-carbohydrate diet might find it healthy if their triglycerides and LDL levels are within the normal range. The positive impact on triglycerides and LDL is outweighed by the health benefits of weight loss.

Humans are adaptable omnivores, historically thriving on a diverse range of food sources. This adaptability means there are numerous ways to maintain a healthy diet.

Three diet plans DASH (Dietary Approaches to Stop Hypertension), Mediterranean, and MIND (Mediterranean DASH Intervention for Neurodegenerative Delay) show promise in promoting heart and brain health while reducing the risk of diabetes. All three emphasize lean meats, fish, whole grains, fruits, vegetables, and olive oil while limiting salt, sweets, and eliminating ultra-processed foods and sugary beverages. Additional information on these diets can be found at the American Heart Association (heart.org) and the National Institute of Aging (nia.nih.gov/health). Plant-based diets (vegetarian and vegan) are also heart-healthy but require supplementation with omega-3 fatty acids, vitamin B12, and possibly other micronutrients like iron. See Appendix B for a summary of these plans.

SPECIFIC NUTRITION GUIDANCE

The idea behind precision nutrition is to create specific dietary recommendations tailored to individual factors such as genetics or the microbiome (bacteria in the intestinal tract). While this concept is intriguing in theory, considering the generally poor quality of the American diet where 38 percent of women aged forty to fifty-nine and 23 percent of women aged sixty and older consume fast food daily it may be more beneficial to focus on implementing proven strategies on a broader scale. Rather than relying on genetic and microbiome testing, which may only be accessible to certain socioeconomic groups, perhaps it is more practical to promote widespread measures that we already know are effective reducing fast food consumption, increasing vegetable and fiber intake, and eliminating sugar-sweetened beverages and fruit juice. Instead of precision nutrition targeting a select few, the emphasis should be on promoting good nutrition for everyone.

9

Supplements Through Menopause

Approximately 60% of adult women in the United States are currently using at least one supplement. While some women take these products for general health or preventive care, others explore various supplements during the menopause transition and post-menopause, seeking relief from symptoms or addressing menopause related concerns referred to as "menoceuticals."

Supplements are increasingly marketed as contributors to wellness, emphasizing achieving a healthy lifestyle from the outside in. However, this ties back to the same strategy used in the 1950s with Premarin—linking products to well-being through lifestyle marketing, which, despite its questionable foundations, proves effective.

Supplements encompass a broad range of over-the-counter (OTC) products, including vitamins, minerals, botanicals, amino acids, hormones, phytoestrogens, fish oils, probiotics, desiccated animal parts, and dietary supplements. Unfortunately, these products are rarely studied and essentially unregulated.

The Dietary Supplement Health and Education Act (DSHEA) passed in 1994 removed multiple safeguards for consumers. Companies are not required to prove that the product contains what is advertised on the label, leading to common occurrences of adulterated products. This can involve substituting the main ingredient for a cheaper alternative, having no active ingredient at all, or even replacing a botanical with a pharmaceutical drug. Instances have been reported where herbal products, including those sold at major retailers, did not contain any of the herbs listed on the labels. The lack of quality control not only jeopardizes consumers who might unknowingly ingest pharmaceuticals or harmful botanicals but also hinders the validity of research studies that rely on uniform and accurately labeled supplements.

In essence, the supplement industry operates on a "buyer beware" principle, with potential risks extending beyond the contents of the product to the integrity of scientific studies. This stands in stark contrast to pharmaceuticals, where there is a level of assurance regarding the accuracy of the prescribed dose.

The supplement industry in the United States faces a notable issue with safety testing these products are assumed safe unless the Food and Drug Administration (FDA) receives evidence of harm. This lack of safety studies comes at a cost, with supplements causing around 23000 emergency room visits annually and contributing to an increasing number of cases of liver failure. Even when the FDA is informed, the response typically involves issuing a mild warning letter for product removal. Given the $30-billion-a-year industry's indifference to such warnings, the lack of testing, coupled with the absence of a research and development pipeline, allows swift replacement of any product pulled from the market. Like shark's teeth, there's always another one.

Supplement advertising regulations are also lenient under the DSHEA, permitting vague "structure/function claims" about body parts and physiology. These claims, such as "maintaining hormone health" or providing "ovary support" or "memory support," can be made without defining the terms or presenting evidence. The industry has thrived since the relaxed regulations in 1994, with the number of supplements on the market growing from 4000 to 55000 by 2012. Medical practitioners often recommend supplements, and financial ties, similar to those with Big Pharma, may exist.

The lack of a database linking providers to financial support from the supplement industry complicates transparency. Some providers sell supplements in their offices, potentially even their own branded ones, creating an imbalance of power and raising ethical concerns. The American College of Obstetrics and Gynecology discourages obstetrician-gynecologists from selling or promoting nonmedical products without adequate evidence and warns against using professional influence to enroll participants in marketing schemes. It emphasizes the importance of avoiding direct sales of medications or devices when alternative vendors exist.

The Women's Health Initiative in 2002 created confusion and fear around estrogens, leaving a gap filled by supplements, similar to bioidentical and compounded hormones. Pre-2002, there were fewer nonhormonal options for menopausal symptoms, leading many women to turn to supplements. Dismissal and disenfranchisement by the medical system also drive women toward supplements, finding validation and understanding in those recommending these alternatives.

However, claims of inherent naturalness in supplements exploit fears about hormones, misleadingly equating natural with safety. In reality, vitamins and minerals are best absorbed from food due to the combination with fiber and other factors enhancing absorption. Whether a substance is found in nature is a matter of marketing, not medicine; the key considerations are indications, safety, and efficacy.

Another issue with supplements lies in their studies, often industry-funded and showing positive effects, though frequently exhibiting poor study design. Low-quality studies with positive results lack meaningful medical conclusions, akin to identifying a person in poor light from a distance an uncertain endeavor yielding minimal information. Despite this confusion, some supplements are medically indicated, such as folic acid preconception, vitamin D for those with insufficient dietary and sun exposure, or multivitamins for individuals with nutrient absorption difficulties, like post-bariatric surgery patients. Certain vegans and vegetarians may need iron and/or vitamin B12 supplements due to the absence of these nutrients in plant-based diets.

Compounding the confusion, headlines from reputable medical sites often make vague claims about the anti-inflammatory properties of vitamins and supplements, creating a misleading impression of their effectiveness.

REVELATIONS OF WOMEN'S CONTRIBUTIONS: MEDICINE, MIDWIFERY, AND PLANT WISDOM

Numerous menopause supplements are rooted in the notion that ancient, once widely known and potent recipes, were suppressed by patriarchal medicine, the pharmaceutical industry, or both. The inclination to idealize the extensive literature on remedies in ancient Egyptian, Greek, Persian, Hindu, and Chinese texts exists, yet many were based on outdated disease models. For instance, in ancient Egypt, a woman with a sore ear and jaw would receive vaginal pessaries and fumigation, a practice inconsistent with contemporary medical understanding. Ancient Greek therapies often revolved around substances thought to be drying, grounded in the belief that women's health problems stemmed from excessive moisture an outdated concept.

Cherry-picking of favourable aspects from ancient therapies is common, as seen in the rebranding of vaginal fumigation in ancient Greece as modern vaginal steaming. However, the reality is that some ancient recipes involved burning a puppy or dog stuffed with herbs to produce steam. Ingredients might also have been chosen for cultural or religious significance, reflecting the worldview of the time. The costliness of certain ingredients may have been intentional, as expensive medications often exhibit a stronger placebo effect, as observed in the historical use of castoreum from beavers in European therapies.

Western medical remedies from the 1500s to the early 1900s were influenced by misconceptions, such as the belief that the absence of menstruation indicated dangerous humours accumulating. Treatments often involved bloodletting or purgatives. Women were thought to have an overly hot temperament, leading to the prescription of sudorifics. Opium, alcohol, and later cannabis were incorporated into remedies, with cannabis suggested in the 1800s to temper the hypersexual nature of menopausal women.

Some claim herbal menopause therapies originate from ancient Chinese medicine, but Charlotte Furth argues that the modern diagnosis of menopause was transferred to traditional Chinese medicine (TCM) from nineteenth-century medicine. TCM historically didn't distinguish menopause from old age, and any TCM recommended for menopause is based on nineteenth-century recipes. Understanding these historical origins is crucial, as some people are drawn to these therapies under the mistaken belief that they are ancient.

Given our current knowledge of phytoestrogens, the effectiveness of ancient recipes containing these plant substances is questioned. Modern phytoestrogen supplements are marginally effective at best, and they contain more active compounds than ancient recipes, making the latter unlikely to have been as effective. It's suggested that ancient plants might have been contaminated with mycotoxins, potent substances produced by fungus with estrogen like activities. If so, the therapy might have worked due to an unknown contaminant rather than the efficacy of the recipe.

Emphasizing the need to scrutinize the medical efficacy and safety of botanicals does not imply dismissal but rather a commitment to understanding the physiological effects and ensuring safety. This approach aligns with feminist ideals, empowering women with accurate information about their health. Historical medicines, once proven effective and safe, have been incorporated into modern medicine. It is a continuous process of exploration and validation of active compounds in nature, ensuring both safety and efficacy. The critical examination of historical medicine is consistent with the rejection of outdated beliefs about women's bodies, aligning with the principles of evidence-based medicine.

DIETARY SUPPLEMENTS: MODERN ALTERNATIVES TO TRADITIONAL PATENT MEDICINES

Exclusive elixirs and mixtures have a long history, initially referred to as nostrum remedium, meaning "our remedy" in Latin, eventually evolving into the term "nostrums." The concept of "patent medicine" originated from products that gained favor with royalty, receiving royal letters or patents as endorsements. These products were extensively promoted with extravagant claims and endorsements from satisfied users, much like many contemporary supplements. The popularity of patent medicines peaked in the 1800s, a time when women approaching menopause often turned to them due to the crude and ineffective nature of prevailing medical therapies, including practices such as bloodletting, leeches to the vulva, and invasive surgeries like ovary removal.

Advertisements for patent medicines were specifically targeted at women, promoting the same product for various medical conditions, from uterine prolapse to infertility, missed periods (coded for pregnancy, suggesting the product's potential to induce abortion), and menopause. Some of these concoctions contained toxic elements like pennyroyal, a mint family herb extract known for its abortifacient properties. Other common ingredients included quinine, boric acid, and the obroma oil, which is recognized as cocoa butter. Surprisingly, certain patent medicines even incorporated chocolate.

One notable success in the realm of patent medicines was Lydia Pinkham's Vegetable Compound, designed for women's ailments, particularly during menopause. Lydia Estes Pinkham created this blend of alcohol, roots, and herbs in her kitchen in 1873. Initially a small venture, Pinkham's business expanded as her product gained popularity. Advertised as "A Woman's Cure for Women's Ills," it claimed to address a myriad of issues, from headaches to depression. However, we now understand that these conditions result from diverse biological processes, and a one-size-fits-all therapy is not feasible.

Each bottle of Pinkham's Vegetable Compound came with an eighty-page book on women's health, and women were encouraged to send in questions for Lydia Pinkham to answer. Pinkham's original recipe contained ingredients like black cohosh, life root, unicorn root, pleurisy root, and fenugreek seed, with black cohosh believed to address menopausal symptoms. The recipe's alcohol content, initially undisclosed, was revealed to be 19.3 percent, equivalent to the alcohol content in most port wines.

In 1911, Pinkham's Vegetable Compound was tested, showing the same alcohol content but no evidence of active substances. A trial of a home version of Pinkham's tonic, focusing on the alcohol part, was conducted, revealing some mild effects on a dull day. Despite this, it's crucial to note that this experiment is not recommended as therapy. The findings suggest that while there might be some active ingredient, it may not align entirely with the advertised claims.

OMEGA 3 SUPPLEMENTS

A substantial clinical trial monitoring over 13000 women aged fifty-five and above revealed that the intake of a 1 g omega-3 supplement, specifically the Omacor brand (a prescription fish oil supplement), led to a 40 percent reduction in heart attacks for White women consuming less than one and a half servings of fish weekly. Remarkably, the reduction was even more pronounced at 77 percent for African American women, irrespective of their fish intake. Omacor, being an FDA-approved prescription, ensured known dosage and purity. While there are vegan omega-3 supplements derived from seaweed, non-prescription options lack the assurance of content and dosage. Adverse effects of a daily 1 g omega-3 fatty acid supplement are infrequent but may include bad breath, heartburn, nausea, diarrhea, headaches, and occasionally malodorous sweat.

Prescription omega-3 fatty acids are employed in higher doses, up to 4 g daily, to address elevated triglycerides. At these levels, they can reduce triglycerides by 20 percent to 30 percent. However, it's important to note that they can influence blood clotting and may interact with anticoagulant medications. Therefore, such elevated doses should be administered only under medical supervision.

For numerous women, incorporating a daily 1 g omega-3 supplement into their routine is a sensible choice.

VITAMIN B12

Vitamin B12 plays a crucial role in the production of red blood cells, maintaining a healthy nervous system, and facilitating various metabolic processes and DNA synthesis. Insufficient levels of vitamin B12 are linked to symptoms such as fatigue, depression, irritability, mouth ulcers, and tingling in the hands and feet. The recommended daily intake of vitamin B12 is 2.4 mcg, and a 3-ounce serving of salmon exceeds that amount, while a cup of milk provides 1.1 mcg. It's important to note that vitamin B12 is not naturally present in plants.

The absorption of vitamin B12 becomes less efficient with age, resulting in approximately 20 percent of individuals aged sixty and older experiencing deficiency. Women aged fifty and older, as well as those following a vegan diet, should closely monitor their vitamin B12 intake and consider supplementation if necessary. Many vegan foods are fortified with vitamin B12, such as certain breakfast cereals, nutritional yeasts, and plant-based milks like soy. Additionally, medications like metformin for type 2 diabetes, acid reflux medications, and weight loss surgery can interfere with vitamin B12 absorption, necessitating supplements in these cases.

While vitamin B12 injections are often portrayed as a remedy for fatigue and are popular in wellness circles, it's essential to recognize that they should only be administered by healthcare providers. The vibrant red liquid may resemble an elixir, but obtaining these injections from a qualified professional is crucial. It's noteworthy that at events like the "goop health" conference, the promotion of intramuscular vitamin B12 injections for wellness is observed. However, these injections should be prescribed by healthcare providers and are only suitable for individuals unable to absorb sufficient vitamin B12 from supplements.

The marketing of vitamin B12 injections as natural, immune-boosting (although scientifically unsupported), and wellness-promoting is contrasted with the skepticism often directed towards other interventions, such as vaccines, labeled as "Evil Pharma." Interestingly, vitamin B12 injections are manufactured by pharmaceutical companies and contain small amounts of aluminum, a component falsely claimed by some to make vaccines unsafe or unnatural. It's crucial to recognize that, although the amount of aluminum in both vitamin B12 injections and vaccines is considered very safe, the frequency of vaccine administration is significantly lower than that of monthly vitamin B12 injections over an extended period.

VITAMIN E

Vitamin E comprises a group of fat-soluble compounds known as tocopherols and tocotrienols, functioning as antioxidants crucial for immune system support and heart health. Deficiency of Vitamin E is exceptionally rare in North America. It can be sourced from various foods, including leafy green vegetables, nuts, seeds, vegetable oils, and fortified cereals. Numerous studies examining vitamin E supplements for preventive health measures have indicated no protective effects against heart disease, cancer, or cognitive decline associated with aging.

Concerns have been raised in some studies regarding vitamin E supplements, indicating a slight but elevated risk of mortality for individuals consuming doses of 400 IU daily and possibly even for those taking as little as 150 IU daily.

NON-PRESCRIPTION HORMONES

Over-the-counter (OTC) hormones are widely available, including platforms like Amazon. It is advisable to steer clear of these products for several reasons beyond potential absence of actual hormones. The following are the four most commonly marketed items for women in the menopause continuum:

- **Progesterone Cream:** Despite claims of containing progesterone, this cream is often ineffective, as it is poorly absorbed (if at all) through the skin. If a woman relies on a progesterone cream while taking estrogen to protect her uterus, she could be at risk for endometrial cancer. Recommending topical progesterone is considered questionable menopause advice.
- **Any Product Claiming to Contain Estrogen:** The quantity of estrogen is crucial for assessing the risk of blood clots and endometrial cancer. Non-pharmaceutical products claiming to contain estrogen may pose safety concerns. For instance, Life Extension's "Estrogen for Women" is misleadingly labeled, as it is a blend of herbal products largely ineffective for menopausal symptoms, despite its suggestive name.
- **Dehydroepiandrosterone and DehydroepiaNdrosterone Sulfate (Dhea and Dhea-S):** Produced by the adrenal gland and ovaries, these hormones are the most abundant steroids in the body. While their functions are not fully understood, they are believed to impact brain function

and inflammation. Some advocate for DHEA during menopause due to its role in hormone production. However, numerous studies—albeit of questionable quality—have found no benefits for sexual function, overall well-being, cognitive function, or effects on lipids or blood sugar. While DHEA proves effective as a prescription-only vaginal therapy for genitourinary syndrome of menopause, there is no evidence supporting its use in menopausal or postmenopausal women or for addressing issues related to desire.

- **Pregnenolone:** Another precursor hormone in the pathway from cholesterol to progesterone, estradiol, and testosterone. A misconception suggests that during times of stress, the adrenal gland redirects pregnenolone to produce stress hormones like cortisol, resulting in a supposed reduction of estradiol and progesterone levels. This phenomenon is commonly termed pregnenolone steal. However, there is no supporting evidence in the medical literature, and the hypothesis lacks biological plausibility based on the body's functioning. While stress can temporarily interrupt menstruation and chronic stressors may impact reproductive function through intricate hormone signaling, this is unrelated to insufficient pregnenolone in the ovaries. The unfounded concept of pregnenolone steal is often linked with another unsubstantiated condition, adrenal fatigue, which posits that stress depletes the adrenal gland. When individuals receive these inaccurate diagnoses, it does not dismiss their symptoms but indicates a misdiagnosis. It is advisable to forego pregnenolone supplements and disregard anyone suggesting the diagnoses of pregnenolone steal or adrenal fatigue.

PROBIOTICS

Probiotics refer to living microorganisms that bring about health benefits to the host, essentially acting as beneficial bugs for the body. In the 1990s, probiotics gained prominence in women's health, initially recommended for the prevention of vaginal and bladder infections. However, their current marketing extends to a broad spectrum of medical concerns and conditions. Despite the buzz surrounding probiotics, there is limited scientific evidence supporting their widespread use in women's health. The gastrointestinal and vaginal microbiomes, which consist of bacterial communities, are intricate, dynamic, and our comprehension of them is in its early stages. The notion that they can be easily manipulated solely for positive benefits with a probiotic pill leans more towards science fiction than scientific fact. Nevertheless, there is data suggesting that probiotics may aid in preventing a potentially harmful type of antibiotic-associated diarrhea known as Clostridium difficile enterocolitis.

For women navigating through the menopause continuum, probiotics are often recommended to prevent urinary tract infections (UTIs) or bladder infections. However, the existing studies are of low quality, and a 2015 Cochrane review, assessing the available evidence, concluded that there was no significant benefit demonstrated for probiotics compared to placebo or no treatment. The data were limited, derived from small studies with inadequate methodological reporting, making it challenging to rule out potential benefits.

Research involving a strain known as Lactobacillus crispatus, a predominant beneficial bacterium in the vagina for many women, indicates a potential to reduce the recurrence of vaginal infections such as bacterial vaginosis. Combining Lactobacillus crispatus with standard therapy for bacterial vaginosis decreased the risk of recurrence from 45 percent to 30 percent. While this could be a helpful addition pending further long-term studies, it is not a comprehensive solution. Notably, this specific probiotic is not currently available over the counter, and the available data for other probiotics and vaginal health is generally unimpressive.

Probiotics encounter quality control issues similar to other supplements. A study found that 33 percent of probiotics had fewer bacterial colonies than claimed on the label, and 42 percent were mislabeled, either lacking the claimed bacteria or containing different species. Additionally, these products are often relatively expensive.

OTHER SUPPLEMENTS

Here are some alternative formulations often marketed to women experiencing menopause:

Antioxidants

These are compounds that may prevent cellular damage caused by free radicals, unstable molecules produced naturally by the body or found in the environment (such as cigarette smoke and sunlight). Examples include vitamins E and C, selenium, and carotenoids found in foods like carrots, pumpkin, and tomatoes. While vegetables and fruits are rich in antioxidants, there is insufficient evidence supporting the use of antioxidant supplements for the general population. Some studies even indicate potential risks, as discussed earlier with vitamin E. For instance, women taking antioxidant supplements during breast cancer chemotherapy faced an increased risk of cancer recurrence. Until quality data emerges, it is advisable to obtain antioxidants from a balanced diet.

Biotin

Also referred to as vitamin B7, often recommended for hair and nails. However, there is no evidence supporting its efficacy unless a person has a biotin deficiency. Abundant in various diets, sources include salmon, egg yolks, and sweet potatoes. Some biotin supplements contain excessively high amounts, as it is a water-soluble vitamin, and the excess is excreted as expensive urine. Elevated biotin levels can interfere with several lab tests, including hormone levels and thyroid tests.

Green Tea Extract

Despite the health benefits of green tea, the extract form has been associated with liver failure, making it an unfavorable choice.

Iodine

Marketed to women over forty for thyroid and immune system support. While nonpregnant adults need 150 μg of iodine per day, readily available in iodized table salt, dairy, eggs, and fish, excessive iodine intake can paradoxically lead to hypothyroidism. Some women consume over-the-counter iodine supplements excessively, developing hypothyroidism. Studies also link excessive iodine intake to autoimmune thyroiditis and papillary thyroid cancer.

Multivitamins

Rebranded for women over fifty, these products have limited benefits for healthy women and may even pose risks. Some studies suggest that the antioxidants in multivitamins may protect cancer cells as well. Excess fat-soluble vitamins may accumulate in fat, potentially causing harm, and high doses may affect the absorption of essential nutrients from food. In general, unless there are specific reasons like weight loss surgery, multivitamins are not recommended.

Vitamin A

Doses exceeding 10,000 IU a day are associated with an increased risk of osteoporosis. Vitamin A deficiency is rare, yet supplements aimed at women often contain such high doses, providing risk without proven benefit. However, topical retinol and prescription vitamin A have demonstrated benefits in reducing wrinkles and promoting collagen growth.

Vitamin B6 and B12

A combination of these vitamins is associated with an increased risk of osteoporosis and fractures, with higher doses correlating with greater risks.

Yam Creams

Capitalizing on the premise that pharmaceutical hormones are derived from diosgenin found in yams. However, the body cannot convert diosgenin into hormones, and yams lack medicinal properties. Topical yam creams claiming benefits like mood balance, adrenal support, and hormone regulation have been shown to offer no real advantages in studies. These products are considered deceptive and a scam, as yams should be regarded as food, not medicine.

CONDUCTING INDEPENDENT RESEARCH

Menopause-focused supplements, or menoceuticals, should undergo the same critical examination as prescription medications. Given the often low quality of research in this field, it is crucial to ask specific questions when considering these products:

How Can This Product Benefit Me In A Meaningful Way?

Reject vague claims like "ovary support" or "adrenal support." Demand clarity regarding expected outcomes and precise dosage information. For instance, a daily intake of 1 g of omega-3 fatty acids has been proven to reduce the risk of heart attacks.

Be Cautious Of Products Promising Universal Benefits:

Conditions like hot flushes, mood swings, cramps, and headaches vary widely, and the notion of a one-size-fits-all remedy lacks biological plausibility. If a supplement seems too good to be true, it probably is, and reputable pharmaceutical companies would have embraced it already.

Consult Medical Professional Organizations' Opinions:

Check recommendations from respected entities such as the North American Menopause Society (NAMS), International Menopause Society (IMS), American College of Obstetrics and Gynecology (ACOG), or the Society of Obstetricians and Gynecologists of Canada (SOGC). Use a search engine to find information on the supplement and its stance from these societies.

Seek Advice From The Office Of Dietary Supplements At NIH:

Visit ods.od.nih.gov to learn about the recommendations from the Office of Dietary Supplements at the National Institute of Health.

Identify Potential Risks, Including Financial:

Unlike prescription drugs, supplements lack detailed product inserts outlining side effects and interactions with medications. Never assume a supplement is harmless. Explore the National Center for Complementary and Integrative Health (www.nccih.nih.gov) for safety information. Also, consult your pharmacist and inform your healthcare provider about supplement usage. Financially, supplements can range from $20 to $90 or more monthly, making it a considerable long-term investment.

Consider Dietary Changes Before Supplements:

Explore dietary adjustments as a potential alternative. Consult a registered dietitian or nutritionist for economical recommendations. In some cases, health insurance may cover these consultations. Even if not covered, a single consultation could pay off quickly, considering the cost of supplements over time.

Assess The Motivations of Those Recommending the Product:

Confirm if the individual recommending the supplement stands to gain financially. Seek advice from a medical professional without any financial interest in the product for unbiased information.

Be Cautious of Terms Like Pregnenolone Steal or Adrenal Fatigue:

If the person recommending the supplement uses these terms, seek a second opinion from another professional.

OPT For Independently Verified Products:

Look for supplements verified by independent agencies for purity. Seals of approval from organizations such as NSF International, US Pharmacopeia (USP), or Consumer Lab indicate that the product has been tested for purity, reducing the risk of adulteration and ensuring that the product contains what the label claims.

10

Bone Health and Injury Prevention

Estrogen, a key female sex hormone, plays a vital role in maintaining bone density and strength. The decline in estrogen levels during menopause can lead to accelerated bone loss, making women more susceptible to osteoporosis and fractures. Osteoporosis is a condition characterized by porous and brittle bones, resulting in an increased risk of fractures, particularly in the hip, spine, and wrist.

Understanding the Impact of Menopause on Bone Health:

OSTEOPOROSIS: UNDERSTANDING THE ISSUE

Bone loss initiates subtly and without symptoms, starting as osteopenia and progressing to osteoporosis, making bones porous, brittle, and prone to fractures. The National Institutes of Health Consensus Conference defines osteoporosis as a condition marked by increased skeletal fragility, low bone density (T-score below –2.5), and microarchitecture deterioration. It's crucial to recognize that this disease can be potentially fatal.

Currently, in the United States, ten million people (eight million women) have osteoporosis, and thirty-four million have osteopenia, affecting 55 percent of the population aged fifty and above. Half of women in this age group will experience an osteoporosis-related fracture in their remaining lifetime, with the number expected to exceed three million by 2025. Hip fractures pose a significant challenge, as only 15 percent of patients can walk unaided after six months, and 24 percent of Americans over fifty with hip fractures may not survive a year. Osteoporosis also raises the risk of wrist and vertebral fractures, causing pain, disability, and disfigurement. Vertebral fractures contribute to the hunched-over posture often seen in elderly women.

By the age of eighty-five, a majority of Caucasian women in the U.S. will have at least one partial spinal deformity. African American and Asian American women face varying risks, with skin pigment influencing bone structure. Men generally have thicker bones due to genetic and testosterone factors, but osteoporosis-related fractures cost the healthcare system around $19 billion annually, estimated to reach $25.3 billion by 2025, with hip fractures representing 80 percent of expenses, averaging $35,000 per patient.

DESIGNED FOR LIFETIME STURDINESS

Contrary to the common belief that aging weakens bones, humans, including postmenopausal women, are inherently designed for lifelong bone strength. Indigenous populations with hunter-gatherer lifestyles and strong connections to the earth, regular exercise, and whole-food diets rarely experience osteoporosis. Our deep connection to the earth influences the health of the first emotional center, linked to a sense of belonging, safety, and security, impacting bones, blood, and the immune system.

In a culture that fosters detachment from our bodies, many women have lost their sense of connection, leading to first-emotional-center diseases like osteoporosis. Factors such as refined-food diets, poor nutrient intake, and sedentary lifestyles contribute to bone loss at increasingly younger ages. Weight-bearing exercise and sunlight, essential for bone health, are explored in this chapter.

BUILDING AND MAINTAINING HEALTHY BONES

To ensure the strength and vitality of your bones, it's essential to comprehend the innate and seamless process through which your body continuously constructs and remodels bone throughout your life. The progression toward osteoporosis is, in fact, a survival mechanism honed over millions of years of evolution to maintain biochemical balance. By aligning with this inherent body wisdom, even weakened bones can regain their strength.

Bone metabolism is an intricate interplay of construction and demolition crews operating side by side. Each of the 206 bones contains cells that deposit a collagen-based protein framework, later fortified by minerals from the blood, forming bone. Simultaneously, cells within bones can break down this structure. In childhood, bone builders outpace bone destroyers as we grow. However, the balance can shift with age due to various factors like depression, vitamin D and mineral deficiencies, a high-acid diet, and steroid use. Such imbalances can lead to weakened bones.

Bones serve as crucial storehouses for essential minerals such as calcium, phosphorous, and magnesium, vital for the proper functioning of every cell in the body. Calcium, for instance, plays a key role in processes ranging from heartbeats to nerve cell firing. When blood calcium levels drop, a cascade of reactions is triggered:

- The parathyroid gland releases parathyroid hormone (PTH).
- PTH stimulates the kidneys to convert stored vitamin D into an active form and releases calcium from bone surfaces.
- Activated vitamin D enhances calcium absorption in the intestine, encourages kidney calcium retention, and facilitates more calcium release from bones.

Once blood calcium levels return to normal, these feedback mechanisms reverse. Similar intricate feedback loops regulate the metabolism of other essential minerals. Osteoclasts, responsible for breaking down bone bits, release over 300 mg of calcium daily. Around 20 percent of adult bone mass is recycled annually, responding to the overall needs of our bodies. A deficit in mineral replacement results in low bone mass.

Bones continually remodel themselves, adapting to physical stress and strain. The osteocyte, a fundamental bone cell, acts as a strain sensor, responding to stress by attracting minerals, a process known as the piezoelectric effect. Regular stress is vital for maintaining strong bones; otherwise, bone loss occurs. Osteoblasts and osteoclasts, the builders and destroyers, communicate through proteins like osteoprotegerin (OPG) and OPG-ligand, with the balance between them determining bone health.

Immune status and bone health are closely linked, both influenced by the first chakra. Diseases like rheumatoid arthritis, lupus, and diabetes often coincide with osteoporosis due to shared bone marrow cells. Chronic infections and autoimmune disorders trigger quiescent T cells to produce OPG-ligand, leading to bone loss. Various factors, including hormone levels, nutritional status, and emotional stress, affect the function of osteoclasts and osteoblasts. Clinical trials exploring synthetic OPG to control osteoclasts and halt bone loss are underway.

Bone Fluctuations Across Lifespan

The development of our skeletal system begins in utero, rapidly expanding through childhood, adolescence, and young adulthood. Peak bone mass, the maximum size and density, is typically reached between twenty-five and thirty years old. Over a lifetime, women may lose 38 percent of their peak bone mass, while men may lose 23 percent. However, some individuals resist bone loss; a study found that 38 percent of men and 2 percent of women aged fifty-five to sixty-four experienced minimal bone loss over eleven years. Despite this, many women start losing bone in their late thirties, preceding the decline in estrogen levels. This loss tends to escalate during perimenopause, with Caucasian women losing 2–4 percent of bone mass yearly in the first five postmenopausal years.

It's crucial to note that healthy women undergoing menopause can experience some bone loss without an increased risk of fractures. Thousands of people with very low bone density do not necessarily face fractures. For instance, in Japan, despite lower hip bone density compared to the United States, hip fracture incidence is significantly lower, even with lower calcium consumption.

The difference between bones prone to fractures and those resilient to them lies in two factors: basic bone architecture and the bone's repair capacity. Osteoporosis may not necessarily lead to fractures, indicating that bone quality and self-repair processes are crucial. Poor bone quality stems from factors like nutritional deficiencies, lack of exercise, insufficient vitamin D, and excessive insulin.

Bone Anatomy

Bones consist of trabecular and cortical bone. Cortical bone forms the protective outer layer, while trabecular bone is spongy and includes marrow. Approximately 80 percent of bone is cortical, and 20 percent is trabecular. Different body parts have varying compositions, influencing susceptibility to bone loss and fractures.

The strength and flexibility of bones depend on the living protein collagen, constituting about 23 percent of bone structure. Collagen provides flexibility, while minerals attached to the collagen matrix create rigidity and strength. Humans and animals are designed to maintain robust bones throughout life, and achieving peak bone mass by the twenties allows for some bone loss without fracture risk as we age. However, modern lifestyles, including lack of exercise, smoking, poor diet, vitamin D deficiency, and eating disorders, often prevent women from reaching peak bone mass by age thirty.

Medical anthropologist Susan Brown emphasizes that bones in Westernized countries are weakening, leading to a widespread decline in bone health. Research comparing historical and modern bone strength reveals that women centuries ago had stronger bones, and Near Eastern populations from 12000 years ago had bone mass nearly 20 percent higher than today.

Beyond strength, body alignment and flexibility contribute significantly to bone health. Proper alignment ensures graceful, pain-free movement, preventing issues in bones and supporting structures. Poor posture, like hunching over, can lead to shoulder, neck, and back problems. Maintaining proper alignment through practices such as Pilates improves posture, flexibility, and overall bone health.

IDENTIFYING OSTEOPOROSIS RISK

Assessing your susceptibility to osteoporosis involves examining the following indicators. If none apply to you, it's likely your bone health is satisfactory, and you can persist with your current healthy lifestyle. However, if multiple factors resonate with you, immediate action is necessary to secure your ability to navigate the future on your feet. Note that some risk factors for osteoporosis also align with those for heart disease, underlining the interconnectedness of bone and heart health.

Family history

If your mother has osteoporosis or experienced osteoporotic fractures, familial predisposition may exist, but proactive measures can mitigate the risk.

Fair complexion

Individuals with fair skin and blue eyes, especially blondes or redheads, tend to have less collagen in bones and skin than those with darker skin tones. This genetic difference affects their bone matrix and mineral deposition.

Body characteristics

Being thin, tall, or having low body fat, especially below 18 percent, can elevate osteoporosis risk. Tall women, particularly with small bones, may face higher risk due to entering menopause with less bone mass.

Smoking

Smoking poisons ovaries, diminishing hormone levels prematurely. Estrogen, testosterone, and progesterone, crucial for bone protection, are affected.

Lack of sunlight exposure

Insufficient exposure to natural sunlight can lead to vitamin D deficiency, vital for healthy bone mineralization.

Sedentary lifestyle

Inactivity hinders weight-bearing exercise essential for bone growth, while studies link bed rest to osteoporosis.

Fitness fanaticism

Excessive exercise, especially with dietary restrictions, can impede mineral intake, disrupt the hormonal feedback loop, and lead to stress fractures, predisposing individuals to osteoporosis.

Amenorrhea history

Irregular periods from excessive exercise or anorexia nervosa disrupt hormone levels, favoring osteoporosis.

Alcohol consumption

Consuming over 25g of alcohol per day interferes with osteoblast and osteoclast function, hindering bone remodeling.

Liver stress

Factors like excessive alcohol consumption, specific medications, and viral hepatitis can stress the liver, crucial for estrogen production, thus affecting bone health.

Caffeine intake

Regular consumption of over two units of caffeine per day increases calcium excretion, potentially leading to significant bone loss over time.

Depression

Chronic depression, associated with high IL-6 levels, stimulates osteoclasts and correlates with abnormalities in hormone levels, increasing osteoporosis risk.

Poor diet

Inadequate intake of fresh foods, leafy greens, and excess junk food can compromise bone health due to nutrient deficiencies.

Premature menopause

Early menopause, surgical ovary removal, or menopause induced by radiation or chemotherapy elevate osteoporosis risk without adequate hormone therapy.

Steroid use

Regular use of steroid drugs accelerates tissue breakdown, including the collagen matrix in bones, and diminishes sensitivity to vitamin D, affecting calcium absorption.

Proton pump inhibitors (PPIs)

Long-term use of PPIs may increase fracture risk by blocking stomach acid production, crucial for nutrient absorption.

Anticonvulsant or benzodiazepine use

These medications may interfere with bone metabolism.

Repeated low bone density scores

Consistent bone density scores more than 2.5 standard deviations below normal in consecutive tests indicate heightened risk.

Height loss

Regular height measurements are crucial, with a significant loss indicating a higher risk for vertebral fractures.

Thyroid disorders

Hyperthyroidism stimulates osteoclast activity, while excess thyroid medication in hypothyroidism may pose a risk. Managing thyroid health is vital for bone health.

Regardless of your risk level, remember that bone is an ever-evolving living structure, offering opportunities for improvement through various interventions, from medications to dietary adjustments.

BONE DENSITY ASSESSMENT

For women with no osteoporosis risk factors, bone density screening is unnecessary. However, those with potential risks should undergo baseline screening, ideally before or during perimenopause. While these screenings don't evaluate bone quality, they quantify bone mass, and low bone mineral density is statistically linked to higher fracture risk, even if fractures typically manifest in one's seventies or eighties. Despite the common delay in insurance coverage until documented osteoporotic fractures occur, investing in preventive measures is crucial.

Heel Bone Density

Utilizing tools like OsteoAnalyzer, heel bone density tests offer an accurate and economical screening method for women of all ages. This method, suitable for baseline screening, is even used for at-risk teenage girls. While less precise than a full DEXA test, heel density tests serve as a valuable early warning system, requiring no prescription and often available at local drugstores.

DEXA Testing

Considered the gold standard, Dual-energy bone densitometry (DEXA) employs low-dose X-rays to measure bone density in the spine and hips. Comparing a woman's bone density to age-specific norms, DEXA categorizes severity based on the deviation from the mean. DEXA, like heel bone density tests, provides a static snapshot, necessitating at least two successive tests six months apart to gauge trends and adjust bone health routines. Testing is available at medical centers, requiring a prescription and preferably the same machine for consecutive readings.

Skin Thickness Testing

Ultrasound measurement of skin thickness, reflecting collagen health, predicts fracture risk as accurately as conventional bone density testing. Combining skin thickness and bone density enhances accuracy. While not widely adopted in the U.S., it's worth inquiring with your doctor about facilities offering this test.

Urine Test for Bone Breakdown Products

Urine tests, like Pyrilinks and Osteomark, measure collagen fragments released during bone breakdown. This provides a day-to-day assessment of bone metabolism, offering early detection before conventional scans identify issues. Available without a prescription, results can be mailed to your home.

The Bottom Line

A strategic combination of bone density screening and urine testing offers a comprehensive approach. Whether using heel density or a DEXA test for baseline assessment, understanding trends requires at least two successive tests. The urine test, revealing immediate bone status, aids in monitoring progress and adjusting bone health strategies. For ongoing stability, annual or biennial urine tests are recommended. These tests empower midlife women to proactively address bone health, preventing further loss and potentially increasing bone density well before osteoporosis symptoms emerge. Creating health becomes a daily endeavor, eliminating the need to wait for symptoms to prompt action.

Hormones and Bone Health

Estrogen supplementation is commonly used to prevent bone loss, although risks associated with Hormone Therapy (HT) prompt consideration of alternative approaches. I recommend prioritizing vitamin D, minerals, exercise, and, if necessary, antiresorptive drugs like Fosamax as primary treatments. If HT is undertaken for other reasons, it effectively safeguards bone health during its course, backed by studies demonstrating a nearly 50 percent reduction in fracture risk with conventional HT. Despite this, maintaining healthy bone mass doesn't mandate estrogen therapy, as women naturally producing even small amounts of estradiol or testosterone exhibit significantly reduced osteoporosis risk.

It's crucial to recognize that hormones are just one facet influencing bone mass. Nearly half of vertebral bone loss in U.S. women occurs before menopause, and certain studies find no significant differences in bone densities between pre/perimenopausal and postmenopausal women. Estrogen's impact on skeletal mass, estimated at 10–15 percent, doesn't solely determine bone health. If estrogen is taken, a minimal effective dose is recommended for bone protection.

Consider hormonal or bone-building interventions if you've experienced:

- History of amenorrhea lasting a year or more
- Premature, surgical, or medical menopause
- History of steroid use
- Strong family history of osteoporosis

Diagnosis of osteopenia or osteoporosis

Remember, hormone therapy or bone-building drugs maintain bone density only while in use, similar to the effects of exercise on bone. If estrogen or androgen use is impractical, natural progesterone, in various forms, could be considered. Synthetic progestin (medroxyprogesterone) stimulates osteoblasts, and low-dose MPA with estrogen prevents fractures, as supported by controlled studies.

Calcium's Role in Bone Health

While high-calcium diets and supplements were traditionally recommended for bone health, recent studies challenge their unequivocal benefits. A Harvard study spanning eighteen years and a meta-analysis involving 170991 women found no conclusive correlation between high-calcium diets and reduced fracture risk. Some experts attribute lower fracture rates in Africa and Asia, despite limited dairy consumption, to factors beyond calcium.

The acidity of blood, influenced by dietary choices, plays a role. Consuming animal protein, grains, and high-glycemic-index foods increases blood acidity, leading to calcium leaching from bones. Eating fruits and vegetables counters this effect. Aim for at least five servings of fruits and vegetables for each serving of animal protein.

While calcium supplements remain beneficial, opt for amino acid-chelated forms like calcium citrate or citrate-malate. A balanced 1:1 or 2:1 calcium-to-magnesium ratio is ideal. Green leafy vegetables provide additional dietary calcium sources. However, relying solely on calcium may overlook the importance of maintaining a balanced diet for bone health. Tums, promoted as calcium supplements, are not recommended due to their antacid nature, lack of magnesium, and potential adverse effects on nutrient absorption.

WHAT ABOUT MEDICATIONS FOR BUILDING BONE?

Often, doctors prescribe newer bone-building drugs as the primary treatment for any woman displaying reduced bone mass, even if osteoporosis or significant osteopenia is not imminent. However, numerous safe and effective alternatives align more naturally with the body's wisdom.

Let's briefly explore commonly prescribed bone-building drugs. Similar to hormone therapy, these drugs exhibit effectiveness only during their use.

Bisphosphonates

Widely prescribed, bisphosphonates are primary postmenopausal osteoporosis treatments. They hinder osteoclast function, preventing bone breakdown, but research suggests potential downsides. Studies link them to severe depression of bone formation and spontaneous fractures. FDA warnings highlight increased risks, especially for atypical femur fractures. While initially praised for reducing fractures by almost 50 percent in osteoporotic women, benefits are limited. Side effects, from bothersome to dangerous, include pain, nausea, and severe esophageal ulcers. Long-term effects remain uncertain, urging cautious use, potentially reserved for older postmenopausal women with major osteoporosis risk factors.

Evista (Raloxifene)

As a Selective Estrogen Receptor Modulator (SERM), Evista has an estrogenic impact on bone but antiestrogenic effects on breast tissue. While beneficial for bone health, it doesn't decrease hip fracture incidence. Concerns include hot flashes and potential dementia risk due to blocking estrogen's beneficial effects on brain cells.

Calcitonin

This peptide regulates osteoclast activity and calcium loss, reducing spinal fracture risk. However, it doesn't impact hip fractures significantly, and bisphosphonates are often deemed more effective. Side effects include nausea and flushing.

In conclusion, individuals with low bone density should prioritize adequate vitamin D, magnesium, and calcium, along with a low-acid diet. Regular weight-bearing exercise is essential. While some might benefit from bisphosphonates, natural methods are preferable as a first-line approach.

GET STRONG

Irrespective of your dietary choices, supplements, or medications, the pivotal revelation is that engaging in weight-bearing exercise, particularly strength training, plays a vital role in establishing and sustaining healthy bones. Sedentary lifestyles contribute significantly to the escalating prevalence of osteoporosis, emphasizing that bone thinning is more a consequence of decreased muscle usage than the natural aging process.

Weight-bearing exercise fosters bone development by stimulating mineralization and remodeling processes. Muscles, connected to bones by tendons, apply force during contractions, influencing bone strength positively. Beyond traditional exercise, practices like yoga and tai chi also enhance bone mass.

However, the benefits extend beyond fortified bones. Participants in weight training programs reported heightened happiness, energy, and self-confidence, showcasing an unexpected positive impact.

Given the multitude of joys and advantages associated with fitness, motivation to embrace strength is essential. Regardless of age or current condition, physical exercise guarantees improvement and a rejuvenated perspective on life. The impact of exercise is so profound that frail nursing-home patients in their late eighties experienced over 100 percent strength increase within ten weeks of a strength-training program. Similarly, elderly patients reduced falls and hospital readmission rates through physiotherapy and vitamin D supplementation.

If such transformations are possible for elderly individuals, envision the potential for a fifty-year-old who commits to a fitness routine. With an average life expectancy of at least eighty-five, possibly a hundred, neglecting muscle and bone health at midlife is a disservice to the promising years ahead. No pharmaceutical, technological breakthrough, or genetic advancement can match the self-derived benefits of staying strong and active. Moreover, regular exercise extends life expectancy by six years, challenging the notion of insufficient time for fitness. Prioritizing exercise is akin to prioritizing daily essentials like brushing teeth or taking a shower, necessitating a shift in mindset. No excuses.

What Would It Take To Get You Moving?

- Reflect on moments of joy from physical activities like dancing, running, or swimming.

- Recollect the last time you experienced the pure pleasure of complete relaxation through activities such as skiing, hiking, or dancing.
- Revisit childhood and teenage activities that brought joy.
- If not exercising presently, assess reasons for abstaining.
- Identify when and why you stopped exercising if applicable.
- Challenge the perception of lacking time for exercise and explore reasons behind it.

EXERCISE FOR VIBRANT HEALTH ON ALL LEVELS

Discovering the right exercise for my body and temperament, independent of family expectations, was a turning point. Regardless of one's fitness past or legacy, vigorous regular exercise becomes imperative for thriving beyond midlife. Exercise sends positive signals, elevating human growth hormone levels, promoting overall vitality. Conversely, sedentary habits convey a message of aging and decline.

Our bodies respond to activity demands. For instance, my mother's Everest trek strengthened her despite past injuries, emphasizing the emotional aspects intertwined with physical health. Consider the activities you want to engage in throughout your life. Personal preferences should guide your choices, ensuring a fulfilling exercise routine.

Case Study: Rony: Couch Potato No More

Rony, fifty-five, sought help for aches, pains, and sleep issues. Despite estrogen use after a hysterectomy, her bone density showed slight loss. Encouraged to adopt an exercise program, Rony started walking, shedding pounds, alleviating discomfort, and improving sleep. Later, she embraced skiing and hiking, making fitness a regular part of her life.

Start Somewhere—Anywhere

For those hesitant about weight training, commit to ten minutes of daily physical activity for thirty days. Simple activities like stretching or dancing can be enjoyable. Movement is contagious, and the initial commitment will likely awaken the inherent desire to move. Even small efforts contribute to the bone-building process.

Seeking Assistance

Once you've established the habit of movement in your life with a month of dancing, consider incorporating resistance training, weight lifting, or Pilates. I recommend seeking guidance from a gym or an adult education class for a personalized strength-training program. This ensures proper technique learning, adaptable for home use later.

The choice between home workouts and a gym depends on your lifestyle and temperament. Each has its advantages and drawbacks. While a gym offers a dedicated fitness environment, home workouts provide convenience. Personally, my fitness routine combines Pilates sessions in a studio, Pilates mat sessions at home, Argentine tango, and regular walks, tailored to my preferences and schedule.

Integrate Strength into Your Daily Routine

To infuse strength training into your daily life, try these exercises during phone calls or spare moments, engaging major muscle groups:

- **Toe Stands:** Stand facing a wall, raising yourself on your toes for three counts. Repeat eight times, gradually increasing the duration.
- **Heel Stands:** Face a wall, raise toes and balls of your feet, balancing on heels for three counts. Repeat eight times, extending the duration.
- **Push-Ups:** Begin with wall push-ups, progressing to floor push-ups gradually. Aim for two sets of eight repetitions.
- **Weights:** Keep a set of dumbbells in front of your TV for biceps curls, overhead presses, rows, or triceps kickbacks during breaks.

Take a gradual approach, respecting your body's cues. Ask your body to breathe deeper and lift more weight over time. Exercise is a discipline, but it becomes enjoyable once you commit to it regularly.

Safe Pilates and Yoga for Women with Bone Loss

Pilates and yoga, with modifications, offer valuable options for women with osteoporosis. Pilates for Buff Bones by Rebekah Rotstein focuses on safe bone-strengthening techniques. Traditional exercises should be adjusted to avoid spinal flexion, enhancing core strength and balance without jeopardizing bone health.

Preventing Joint Pain

Joint problems during perimenopause can be addressed through maintaining range of motion with Pilates, yoga, or the Core Program by Peggy Brill. Emotional aspects affect joint health, and exercises allowing emotional release contribute to holistic well-being. Acknowledging the emotional connection to physical issues, such as frozen shoulder or back pain, opens avenues for healing. Movement is crucial, and understanding the emotional basis enhances the healing process.

THE SUNLIGHT-BONE HEALTH LINK

Amidst warnings about sun exposure dangers, particularly the risks of premature aging and skin cancer, it's crucial to recognize the nuanced relationship between sunlight and bone health. The emphasized risks, although documented, are often exaggerated, especially for individuals in northern climates where sunlight is less intense for most of the year. Women post-menopause, residing above a line approximately from Boston through Chicago to the California-Oregon border, experience a winter-related bone mass loss of 3–4 percent. Even on a sunny December day in northern Maine, adequate ultraviolet exposure for vitamin D production requires exposing a significant portion of the skin to sunlight, an uncommon practice.

The significance of sunlight lies in its ability to facilitate vitamin D synthesis, a hormone crucial for calcium absorption in bones. The key is moderation, as vitamin D deficiency poses risks, such as osteoporosis, beyond just preventing rickets. Adequate vitamin D levels offer various health benefits, from decreasing hypertension to slowing osteoarthritis progression.

Sunlight vs. Vitamin D Supplements

While our bodies evolved to obtain vitamin D from the sun, ancestral habits of sun exposure contrast with modern lifestyles. Outdoor sunlight exposure remains a more reliable predictor of vitamin D levels than dietary intake, which poorly correlates with blood vitamin D levels. Unlike supplements, sun exposure has a built-in mechanism, preventing excessive vitamin D production.

Routine sun exposure without sunscreen for about 20-30 minutes three to five times weekly during sunny months is a natural way to maintain bone mass. The body can stockpile vitamin D for low-sunlight periods. However, efficiency decreases with age, requiring longer exposure for those over sixty-five. A rule of thumb: if sunlight causes skin reddening, it likely contains enough UVB rays for vitamin D synthesis.

Balancing Sun Safety and Health

Harnessing sunlight's benefits requires regular outdoor activities. Small amounts of UVB light yield striking benefits. Recommendations include 10-20 minutes of daily sun exposure without sunscreen, especially for those with darker skin. Early morning or late afternoon sunlight is safest, avoiding midday sun and sunburn. Other methods, such as driving with windows down or creating a sunroom, offer additional vitamin D enhancement.

When Sunlight is Insufficient

In the absence of sunlight, vitamin D must be obtained from the diet. While supplements can help maintain bone mass, they are less reliable than sunlight. Dosages of 2,000–5,000 IU per day are suggested, with higher initial doses under a doctor's supervision. Fortified foods like milk may not provide sufficient vitamin D due to processing issues. Checking vitamin D levels through a blood test is crucial, aiming for 40–100 ng/ml for optimal health.

Tanning Salons and Antioxidants

Tanning salons, despite dermatologists' concerns, can be considered for those at high risk for osteoporosis, depression, or certain cancers, provided overexposure is avoided. Antioxidants, including vitamins E and C, proanthocyanidins, and beta-carotene, help protect the skin from sun damage. Caution is necessary with drug-induced sun sensitivity, as several common medications increase susceptibility to sunburn. Checking with a pharmacist is advisable.

11

Managing Sleep And Recovery

IMPROVING YOUR SLEEP

In the midst of menopause, women often undergo alterations in their sleep patterns, akin to the changes experienced during adolescence. The spectrum of sleep-related challenges is diverse, with some women finding themselves requiring more sleep than ever before, others grappling with insomnia, and yet others realizing that the quality of their sleep has diminished.

Regrettably, insomnia compounds the challenges of the entire midlife transition. Inadequate sleep leads to elevated levels of corticosteroids and catecholamines, stress hormones that, over time, can disrupt hormonal equilibrium and compromise the immune system. Research indicates that between 20 to 40 percent of women contend with sleep disorders, and post the age of thirty-five, women are markedly more susceptible to insomnia compared to men. Furthermore, perimenopausal women often find themselves needing more sleep than their male counterparts of the same age.

Sleep is a crucial mechanism for restoring both physical and mental energy. Notably, experiments with animals have demonstrated that sleep deprivation can lead to fatal outcomes. Inadequate sleep manifests itself in overt drowsiness, fatigue, and irritability. Additionally, cognitive functions suffer, evidenced by decreased concentration, diminished efficiency, lowered work motivation, and a higher incidence of errors in judgment. The stringent sleep requirements imposed by the Federal Aviation Administration on flight crews underscore the importance of adequate sleep in minimizing the risk of accidents. Sleep deprivation can induce "micro-sleeps," brief lapses in attention that may go unnoticed by those in our vicinity. Research also underscores the vital role a good night's sleep plays in maintaining healthy blood pressure levels.

Beyond the immediate effects on alertness and cognitive function, sufficient sleep is closely tied to maintaining a healthy weight. It is not uncommon for individuals to experience a weight loss of two to three pounds or more after a restful night's sleep. In fact, a 2005 study conducted at Columbia University revealed a direct correlation between sleep duration and obesity. Subjects who consistently slept four hours or less per night were 73 percent more likely to be obese than those who slept between seven to nine hours. Those with five hours of sleep faced a 50 percent higher likelihood, and individuals with six hours of sleep had a 23 percent increased risk of obesity. Researchers attribute this to the impact of sleep on hormones—less sleep tends to reduce the production of leptin, the hormone signaling satiety, while increasing the production of ghrelin, the hormone associated with hunger. Consequently, insufficient sleep leaves individuals feeling both hungrier and less satisfied, contributing to weight management challenges.

Insomnia Frequently Communicates Messages From Our Inner Guidance

Insomnia often serves as a communication channel from our inner selves during the transformative phase of menopause. The intertwining of unprocessed emotions such as anger, sadness, or anxiety with the profound changes that accompany midlife often manifests in disrupted sleep patterns and persistent fatigue. The neurochemical landscape crucial for sleep undergoes shifts in many women during menopause, and these changes are intricately entwined with our emotional states.

Consider the scenario where emotional exhaustion persists even after a seemingly sufficient ten-hour sleep following a dispute with a spouse. This exhaustion is not merely a result of physical restlessness but is rooted in the emotional turmoil experienced. A case in point involves a patient who identified the link between her chronic insomnia and her constant worry about her daughter's struggle to establish a career and independent living. The breakthrough came when she made a decision to stop enabling her daughter's dependency by insisting on her finding employment and learning to support herself.

Another patient in the perimenopausal stage found herself perplexed by sleep difficulties, despite the absence of hot flashes, sweats, coffee consumption, or significant stressors. When questioned about her sleep quality when not sharing a bed with her husband, she acknowledged a noticeable improvement. This revelation served as a significant clue from her inner wisdom. Acknowledging this connection, however challenging, became imperative. While I refrained from prescribing a specific solution regarding her sleeping arrangements, I emphasized the importance of remaining aware of this link. Proposing a temporary separation could provide valuable insights into her husband's response and potentially pave the way for deeper intimacy in the future. The acknowledgment of these subtle cues from within can serve as a catalyst for understanding and addressing sleep problems during menopause, leading to a more holistic approach to well-being.

How Long We Sleep To Feel Better?

Our intrinsic biological rhythms bear the brunt of the demands imposed by modern life on our sympathetic nervous system, responsible for keeping us alert. It's easy to overlook the fact that the electric lightbulb is a relatively recent addition in evolutionary terms, and our bodies were not designed to burn the midnight oil routinely. Cultural disdain is often directed towards napping, sleeping in on gloomy mornings, or retiring at sunset. Instead, we celebrate hyperactive individuals who pride themselves on working sixteen-hour days, even boasting about their minimal sleep.

During my medical school days, especially post-lunch lectures, I daydreamed about having a bed on the podium to catch up on sleep while enduring lengthy talks. Some of my fatigue was attributed to low blood sugar from an excessive carbohydrate intake. However, even with an improved diet, sustaining alertness on merely five to six hours of nightly sleep was impossible. Personal experiences of insufficient sleep left me feeling groggy in the morning, struggling to find motivation for my tasks. When life places additional demands on us, it's crucial to be adaptable and compassionate toward our needs. In such moments, what we genuinely require is to retreat to bed, allowing our parasympathetic nervous systems to restore us. Despite societal disapproval, midday naps can be remarkably revitalizing, with some corporations noticing increased employee productivity when nap breaks are permitted.

Sleep, often underrated, is a fundamental bodily function, as vital as breathing and eating. It serves as the most effective means for the body to metabolize excess stress hormones and inflammatory chemicals, mitigating the risk of chronic degenerative diseases such as high blood pressure, arthritis, and cancer. Beyond physical restoration, sleep is essential for memory consolidation and learning, helping us process and integrate daily experiences. A good night's sleep facilitates the integration of new information or skills acquired the day before.

Research indicates that our most restful sleep occurs when we align with our internal biological rhythm. This may involve waking up with the sun and retiring early, typically between nine and ten at night. Discovering your natural rhythm requires discipline, yet it is essential for optimal well-being. Many menopausal women find their previously sufficient sleep inadequate, realizing the increased need for rest. Personally, I observed a heightened need for sleep during perimenopause, acknowledging it as my body's way of seeking restoration amidst life's changes. Both adolescence and perimenopause dictate a biological truth: the necessity for more sleep than at other life stages. It is imperative for women to recognize and honor this need, seeking the rest they require, which may amount to eight to ten hours a night. In times of travel or stress, extended sleep of ten to twelve hours is not uncommon, without any accompanying guilt.

Tips For Improving Sleep During Perimenopause

Enhancing sleep quality during perimenopause requires a personalized approach, acknowledging that what works for one person may not work for another. Engage in a bit of trial and error as you explore various sleep aids, such as meditation, deep relaxation exercises, listening to soothing music, or enjoying a warm mug of chamomile tea. Regardless of your chosen routine, it's crucial to avoid succumbing to "performance anxiety." Refrain from dwelling on concerns about the number of hours of rest you might miss if sleep doesn't come immediately. Resist the temptation to check the clock, and, most importantly, steer clear of allowing your mental to-do list to hijack your bedtime. Avoiding such pitfalls prevents the establishment of night-owl habits that can be challenging to break in the long run.

- **Managing Hot Flashes:** Combatting hot flashes and night sweats takes precedence as they are primary culprits for sleep disruption during menopause. Neurotransmitter changes in the brain, triggered by erratic estrogen levels or imbalances between estrogen and progesterone, often contribute to these symptoms. Maintaining hormonal balance, especially through the calming effects of progesterone on the central nervous system, is crucial. Sleep disturbances caused by hot flashes can be alleviated through natural progesterone cream, estrogen replacement, acupuncture, or herbal remedies. It's important to recognize that unresolved stress and anxiety can exacerbate hot flashes.

- **Cooling Techniques:** Simple measures, such as using a cold pillow like the Chillow, can be remarkably effective in cooling hot flashes. The Chillow, a water-filled foam pillow, naturally dissipates heat, ensuring a cool and comfortable night's sleep. This not only aids in preventing hot flashes from waking you up but also contributes to an overall more restful sleep.
- **Dietary Choices:** Maintaining stable blood sugar and insulin levels is essential for quality sleep. Foods rich in phytoestrogens like soy or supplements such as Pueraria mirifica, can promote a good night's sleep. Avoid going to bed on a full stomach to prevent gastric reflux. Opt for a carefully chosen snack high in protein or complex carbohydrates before bedtime, avoiding refined and processed foods, which hinder rest and relaxation. Antioxidant supplements taken twice a day can further support refreshing sleep.

- **Caffeine and Alcohol:** Minimize caffeine intake, as even one cup of coffee in the morning can disrupt nighttime sleep. Caffeine clears more slowly from the system in women than in men, and it acts as a bladder irritant, leading to nocturnal awakenings. Similarly, limit alcohol consumption, as while it may act as a sedative, it disrupts the brain-stem sleep mechanism, resulting in rebound insomnia.
- **Regular Exercise and Relaxation Techniques:** Regular exercise, apart from its various benefits, improves the ability to achieve restful sleep. However, avoid vigorous exercise within three to six hours of bedtime, as it can stimulate the central nervous system, making it harder to sleep. Relaxation exercises, such as hatha yoga and meditation, can be especially helpful. Experiment with winding down activities in the hour or two prior to bedtime to find what suits your body's response.
- **Optimizing Sleep Environment:** Ensure a dark sleep environment, free from electric lights, passing car headlights, or moonlight streaming through windows. If pure darkness is challenging to achieve, use blackout shades and avoid being able to read the face of your alarm clock, as this can induce anxiety. Consider using an eye pillow scented with calming lavender oil for added comfort in situations where achieving complete darkness is not possible.

Reversing the Impact of Electromagnetic Pollution with Vitamin G (Ground)

Electromagnetic pollution, arising from the surplus of electromagnetic frequencies emitted by everyday appliances like microwave ovens, cell phones, televisions, and computers, can detrimentally affect our health. The clash between these frequencies and our body's low-frequency bioenergetic fields is particularly problematic, leading to various issues, with insomnia being a significant consequence. In susceptible individuals, electromagnetic pollution may also contribute to headaches, arthritis pain, anxiety, and even arrhythmia. Those most at risk are children, the elderly, and individuals with compromised immune systems.

One effective method to counteract electrical pollution is to reconnect with the Earth physically. The Earth's surface contains free-flowing electrons continually replenished by solar radiation and lightning, offering a health-giving electric signal that helps maintain our bodies in a state of bioenergetic balance. Unfortunately, modern life often disconnects us from the Earth due to the prevalence of rubber-and plastic-soled shoes and the shift away from sleeping directly on the ground, as our ancestors once did. Electropollution significantly exacerbates this disconnection issue.

However, the solution is readily available just beyond your doorstep. Walking barefoot on dirt, sand, or grass allows you to electrically ground yourself. For those experiencing insomnia, minimizing cell phone usage and ensuring the unplugging of cordless phones, TVs, and other electrical appliances, including lamps, during the night can be beneficial.

Additional Strategies for Improved Sleep

- **Covering Bedroom Mirrors:** According to the principles of feng shui, mirrors in the bedroom can disrupt sleep by making individuals feel uneasy. To counteract this, cover bedroom mirrors at night or consider their removal. Mirrors can be draped with curtains during the day and drawn back at night to create a more soothing sleep environment.
- **Establishing a Sleep Ritual:** Developing a consistent going-to-sleep ritual, rooted in good sleep habits, is essential for optimal rest. This practice, known as "good sleep hygiene," involves counting backward from the preferred wake-up time to set a regular bedtime. Changing into comfortable attire and completing pre-sleep bathroom rituals half an hour before bedtime signal to the body that it's time to wind down.
- **Limiting Stimulating Activities:** Avoid engaging in stimulating activities such as web surfing, reading disturbing content, or watching the news before bedtime. Disconnecting from electronic devices and removing the television from the bedroom supports relaxation, allowing the parasympathetic nervous system to function optimally.

- **Managing Emotional Stress:** Steer clear of emotionally stressful discussions or challenging phone calls near bedtime. Recognize individual responses to unresolved issues and decide consciously on an approach that works best for personal well-being.
- **Addressing Mental Overactivity:** Combat the common sleep detractor of incessant mental activity by utilizing relaxation techniques. Herbal tinctures like Amantilla and Babuna, warm baths, and engaging in a calming book can help soothe the mind. Consciously infusing bedtime with positive intentions and avoiding clock watching contribute to a more tranquil sleep experience.
- **Putting Worries to Rest:** A useful strategy involves writing down concerns before bedtime and entrusting them to a higher power. This practice helps shift perspective and instills confidence that solutions will emerge after a restful night's sleep.
- **Optimizing Sleeping Surface:** Investing in a supportive mattress is crucial for quality sleep. Considering that we spend about one-third of our lives asleep, replacing mattresses every ten years, or ideally every five, ensures adequate support and promotes overall well-being.

Exercise Caution with Prescription Sleep Medications

When it comes to prescription sleep medications, a word of caution is in order. Health care practitioners often prescribe drugs like Lunesta and Ambien quite liberally, with Ambien ranking as the seventeenth most commonly prescribed drug in 2008. Another category of sleep medications falls under benzodiazepines, including diazepam (Valium), lorazepam (Ativan), and temazepam (Restoril). While these medications act on the GABA receptors in the brain to induce a calming effect, they carry significant risks. All of them are habit-forming, and their effectiveness diminishes over time as the brain develops tolerance, leading to an escalating need for dosage to achieve the same outcome. It's not uncommon to encounter older women who, having been initially prescribed Valium for anxiety and insomnia during perimenopause, find themselves still grappling with addiction thirty years later. While these drugs have their place, it's crucial not to rely on them for extended periods—limit use to seven to ten consecutive days. They may, however, prove useful for those struggling to sleep on overnight flights.

In addition to benzodiazepines, certain antidepressants, such as selective serotonin reuptake inhibitors (SSRIs) like fluoxetine (Prozac), venlafaxine (Effexor), and sertraline (Zoloft), can initially provide relief for sleep problems. However, similar to benzodiazepines, their effectiveness may diminish over time.

Over-the-counter sleep remedies, including diphenhydramine found in products like Sominex or Benadryl, present yet another option. These drugs interfere with the production of acetylcholine, a crucial brain chemical for memory. It's essential to be mindful of the potential long-term consequences, as extended use of these over-the-counter remedies has been linked to serious memory problems and confusion.

While prescription and over-the-counter sleep medications may offer temporary relief, the risks associated with their prolonged use underscore the importance of exploring alternative strategies for managing sleep problems during menopause. Integrative approaches, lifestyle modifications, and natural remedies can provide viable alternatives, minimizing dependence on medications with potential long-term repercussions. It is crucial for individuals to make informed choices about sleep interventions, considering both short-term benefits and long-term consequences for their overall well-being.

Exploring Natural Aids for Restful Sleep

In the pursuit of restful sleep during menopause, the realm of natural sleep aids offers a diverse range of alternatives, steering clear of potential side effects associated with conventional medications. Delving into these options with informed choices can bring about a soothing reprieve. Here's a comprehensive exploration of some noteworthy natural sleep aids:

- **Natural Progesterone:** Consider incorporating ¼ tsp (20mg) of 2 percent natural progesterone skin cream at bedtime. This natural progesterone engages with the GABA receptors in the brain, inducing a calming effect. Reports of addiction to its brain effects are exceptionally rare, with only one case observed in over two decades of practice.

- **Amantilla and Babuna: Derived from the valerian plant and** the flower of the manzanilla plant (commonly known as chamomile), Amantilla and Babuna serve as potent natural medicines. In a controlled study, where patients received 15 drops of each or a combination before sleep, Amantilla demonstrated 82.5 percent effectiveness, while Babuna exhibited 68.8 percent effectiveness. Taking Babuna (15 drops) before sleep, followed by Amantilla (15 drops) just before turning off the lights, can be a valuable ritual for those dealing with anxiety or heightened stress. These tinctures are particularly appealing due to their lack of side effects.
- **Valerian:** Valerian, when compared to small doses of benzodiazepines and barbiturates, has proven equally effective in inducing sleep and preventing nighttime awakening, all without causing morning sleepiness. To bypass its rather unpleasant taste, it is recommended to take valerian in capsule form. A dosage of 150–300 mg of a product standardized to 0.8 percent valerenic acid at bedtime is advisable.
- **Melatonin:** Melatonin, a hormone produced by the pineal gland in response to light and darkness cycles, aids in inducing drowsiness. It also serves as an antioxidant, playing a role in preventing degenerative illnesses. Supplemental melatonin is beneficial for conditions such as depression, shift work, seasonal affective disorder, and jet lag. The typical dose ranges from 0.5–3.0 mg, taken an hour before bedtime. Shift workers can maintain a regular

sleep pattern by taking melatonin an hour before sleep, even during daytime hours. Moreover, melatonin helps reset the biological clock when adjusting to a new sleep/wake cycle.

- **HTP:** The precursor molecule to melatonin, 5-HTP (5-hydroxytryptophan), proves effective in treating sleep disorders, PMS, and seasonal affective disorder. It is generally considered safe and widely available. The initial dose is typically 100 mg three times per day, which can be gradually increased over several months to 200 mg three times per day.

It's worth noting that even natural substances like valerian and natural progesterone may experience diminished effectiveness over time, as they target the same brain receptors as prescription sleep drugs. Therefore, it is advisable to use them sparingly, preferably after exploring alternative routes to achieving a restful night's sleep.

CONCLUSION

You've reached the finish line of this book, but remember, your journey as an athlete is an enduring, dynamic story. Menopause marks the beginning of a new challenge, an adventure that unfolds as a remarkable chapter in your athletic journey. It's a chapter filled with vibrant experiences, potential, and an unwavering spirit.

As you close this book, do so with the understanding that this isn't the end; it's the commencement of something extraordinary. The menopausal transition isn't a signal to slow down, but an opportunity to redefine your capabilities and harness new strengths.

Your athletic journey is a narrative of determination, triumph, and ceaseless growth. It's a story that transcends age and stages, and one that's been enriched with every mile run, every goal scored, and every personal best achieved. Menopause is the next challenge, the next race, and the next summit to conquer.

The finish line of this book is merely the starting line of your next incredible chapter. As you turn the page and continue on your menopause journey, know that the most thrilling and fulfilling moments in your athletic story are yet to come. Keep going, keep believing, and keep writing the story of your life with the indomitable spirit of an athlete.

DISCLAIMER

The information provided in this book is intended for general informational purposes only and should not be considered as medical advice. It is not a substitute for professional medical diagnosis, treatment, or personalized care. Before starting any new health or exercise program, especially if you are experiencing symptoms related to menopause, it is crucial to consult with a qualified healthcare professional or your primary care physician.

Individuals vary, and what may be suitable for one person may not be appropriate for another. This book does not guarantee specific results and is not responsible for any adverse effects or consequences resulting from the use or application of the information presented herein.

Furthermore, the author is not liable for any errors or omissions in the content of this book or for any actions taken in reliance thereon. The reader should independently verify any information provided in this book and consult with their healthcare provider to address their specific health needs and concerns.

Printed in Great Britain
by Amazon

38574341R00096